THE
ILLNESS OF MEDICINE
EXPERIENCES OF CLINICAL PRACTICE

Michael J. Young, M.D.

Published in the United States by GM Books, Beverly Hills, California.

Library of Congress Cataloging-in-Publication Data

Michael J. Young, M.D. "The Illness of Medicine"

Copyright © 2018 by Michael J. Young.

No part of this publication may be reproduced, distributed, or transmitted in any form or by any means, including photocopying, recording, or other electronic or mechanical methods, or by any information storage and retrieval system, without prior written permission from I.P.A. Graphics Management, Inc., dba GM Books, except for brief quotations embodied in critical reviews and certain other noncommercial uses permitted by copyright law. For permission requests, write to the publisher, addressed "Attention Permissions Coordinator," at the address below:

GM Books
269 S. Beverly Dr. #1054 Beverly Hills, CA 90212
(310) 923-2157
www.gmbooks.com

ISBN Print # 978-1-882383580

Digital #978-1-882383597

Cover and Book Design: Michelle Manley, Graphique Designs

Editor: Jon R. Zobenica, former senior editor at The Atlantic Monthly

Printed in the USA

DISCLAIMER: This work contains my personal observations and recollections over the course of my 33 years as a physician. It is intended to create a dialogue and assessment of the delivery of medical services and improve the profession. Over this time, I have witnessed medicine morph from a more principled profession into a business operation. One that is driven by the goal of maximizing revenue while navigating insurance interference, and experiencing a change in the quality and costs of those services. I have tried to recreate events, locales and conversations from my memories of them. No specific persons or places have been named and no observations or comments are directed toward any person or place. The criticisms made and opinions expressed are my own. I have no intent to harm any individuals or institutions.

Dedicated to Robert and Roberta

CONTENTS

	Acknowledgements	i
	Introduction	iii
1	Why a surgeon?	1
2	Medical school	7
3	Residency	15
4	How Things Have Changed	31
5	Injectable Erections	51
6	Technology	57
7	The Seventh Floor	65
8	The Hospital Room	73
9	Viagra, and Things	81
10	Vasectomy	91
11	The Fractured Testicle	97
12	Getting to the Office	103
13	So, You Need Surgery	113
14	Emergencies	145
15	Medical Marketing	153
16	Mistakes	163
17	Cancer	175
18	The Incentive for Payment	185
19	Fearing for Humanity	193
20	Responsibility	199
21	The Legal Mess	203
22	Building a Practice	213
23	Meeting in the Doctors' Lounge	219
24	Nobody Can Do Anything	225
25	First Case, Last Case	235
26	Time to Stop	241
27	How Do We Get Out of This Mess?	251
	Epilogue	261

ACKNOWLEDGEMENTS

In writing this book about my 33 years of experiences and perspectives in medicine, it is impossible to name all of those who, in one way or another, contributed to my understanding of what being a physician means, and what has evolved in the practice of medicine today. The many teachers who have taken the time and energy to guide my learning, and stimulate my educational growth are countless. I thank all who have taught me over the years. From the earliest experiences with my father, to the myriad of professors and physicians who steered me in the proper direction regarding what to do and when to do it, I am forever grateful.

But just as important, I wish to thank the many patients I have had the privilege to treat. People who have entrusted me with their health, who have allowed me to be a part of their lives. It has been stated that a doctor does not treat his first patient the same as his last. We learn along the way, we try to improve our outcomes. I am indebted to the many patients who allowed me to practice my profession along the way. I sincerely hope that I have made many lives better as a result of my involvement.

I would like to thank my friend Jack Conaty for his encouragement to write this book. He was the catalyst to get things going. Dean Maragos, while endlessly practicing his golf swing out of a bunker, afforded me the opportunity to discuss with Ken Pavichevich my intent to get my book out. Kenny in turn, introduced me to my publisher, William Dorich at GMBooks. Thank you, Bill, for your interest and expertise in making this happen. Bill in turn, brought me to my editor Jon Zobenica. Thank you, Jon, for helping my thoughts become expressed more clearly. To Michelle Manley, thank you for contributing your graphic skills in helping to design the creative book cover. Events in life really do run in a circle. My thanks to Bill Niro for his knowledge and patience, as he clarified literary law to me. I am so very appreciative and proud to have all of you as my friends, and in helping me to ascend to my achieving this goal.

To Barbara for her guidance and reviews, and keeping me on track. To Jimmy, for showing me how a superb doctor practices medicine. To my extended family and friends for their support. And finally, to Mom and Dad. You once told me I could do anything for a living, as long as I received my M.D. first. I am so very proud that you did. I couldn't have done any of it without your love and unwavering support.

INTRODUCTION

I want to begin by stating this is not a book about medicine. It is not a description of how to be a patient, or how to be a doctor. It is not about the evolution of medical understanding or of medical science. It is a true-life story of how the medical profession was experienced from my vantage point, from the early days of trying to embrace my father's medical realm to a more recent understanding of where the practice of medicine has gone. It is a recollection of events that help illustrate what has transpired in the *practice of medicine* over the past thirty years or so. I share this perspective not for the reason of criticism or complaint. My goal is to provide an anecdotal point of view while lending commentary to what occurs behind the closed doors of the medical world. As patients, we are frightened to have a medical problem. Something is wrong and in need of repair. We can't do it ourselves, so we must trust somebody else to tend to our most precious commodity: our own body. Nothing else in life will ever come close to the significance of having and maintaining good health. It truly is everything. So how do we know which doctor to see, what hospital to go to, and how to navigate our current-day labyrinth of medical care?

The Illness of Medicine

To be a patient requires only one thing: having an illness. To be a patient who has the illness taken care of properly requires much more than just a good doctor. It requires patience, perseverance, and an understanding of the *system*—a system that in many ways has gotten dysfunctional and out of control; a system that has been taken over by a complex corporate bureaucracy more interested in profit than in actual patient care; a system entangled in a plethora of insurance-company rules and regulations. Most important, the patient is now subject to a problem that can sometimes be nearly as significant as the illness itself: a frightening lack of control over decisions related to one's own health care.

Medical treatment is overly dependent on the managed flow of money within the system. The skyrocketing costs of drugs and treatment, and the bureaucratic restrictions placed on the patient at a time when he or she is most in need and least able to manage the situation, are derelictions in and of themselves. The loss of the patient-doctor relationship requires evaluation and discussion, as do changes in how doctors actually treat their patients today.

This is why I retired from the practice of medicine. It was not out of anger but, rather, because of the frustration with what we—all of us, the patient, society, and the doctors—have allowed to happen to our health-delivery system.

For me, practicing medicine was both an honor and a privilege, something that for nearly thirty years I did to the very best of my abilities. It helped to shape my life and allowed me to study and do what most interested me. Through the practice of medicine, I met literally tens of thousands of patients over the years. I did my very best to help improve their lives in whatever capacity I could. From taking care of the most trivial of problems to managing life-threatening cancer, the practice of medicine engulfed me. I like to think I did it well. However, the business of medicine today is in absolute chaos—something that patients, with their inherent vulnerability, should not have to navigate. Being a medical provider, too, has never been more complicated, or more disappointing and difficult. Many of my previous colleagues simply want to throw in the towel given the absurdities now visited upon the profession.

In the pages ahead I will explore both what has happened in the practice of medicine and possibly how to fix it. The events described in this book are accurate and real. But before we can find a repair to the problem, we need to understand what, along the way, helped create the mess in the first place. Just as concerning is that resolving the problem may take the same amount of time that the problem itself took to develop. For if the current problem of how we deliver medical care was socially induced, realignment and improvement will likewise occur only if we work together to change our perspective. If we eliminate the legal straitjacket medicine finds itself in, address the excess profits sought by the pharmaceutical and medical-product industries, and make health insurance affordable and *functional*, improvement in health care delivery may actually occur. Are these events even possible? Perhaps not. Perhaps they're so socioeconomically ingrained in our culture that only an idealist would think such a dysfunctional system could be modified and improved.

Let's look at the problems—up front and in a very personal manner. Perhaps then we may begin to understand the direction we need to go in order to fix our medical care.

CHAPTER 1

Why a Surgeon?

I recall as a teenager having the opportunity to observe surgery. My father invited me to come with him to the hospital one summer day to watch what he did for a living. I vividly remember the excitement of walking down the hallway with him toward the operating rooms. There was a peculiar odor in the hallway: one of absolute cleanliness. The floors appeared to glisten as they reflected back the fluorescent ceiling lights. The walls, floor, and ceiling were a very crisp, clean white—just as I had seen on television and in the movies. As we pushed through the double doors into the reception area of the operating room, I felt as though we were entering a sanctuary. It was very exciting.

This was in the mid-1970s. The nurses in the community hospital where he performed his ophthalmological surgery were wearing their nursing caps—the styles of which were reflective of their nursing schools and degrees. The nurses wore white nylons. Their shoes were white, as were their skirts and blouses. Everything appeared clean and sterile. I remember how intimidated I felt not knowing where exactly to stand, what to say (if anything), or how

CHAPTER 1 | The Illness of Medicine

to appear. Unlike in my day-to-day experiences, here everyone seemed to have a specific role, a specific code of behavior—one that I was able to observe but that I didn't quite understand.

The nurses greeted us and addressed my father as "Doctor." It was so formal. I remember my father appearing to me as larger than life—on a different plane from everyone else in the room. He was the Doctor, in charge and in command, and he was treated with absolute respect by those in attendance.

We then proceeded to the "Doctor's Locker Room" to change into scrubs. (There would be more than one such locker room today, labeled either "Men's" or "Women's." But back then, nearly all doctors were men, and nurses were most often women.) I recall that having entered this sanctum within the hospital, I felt I'd become part of a special group of people. Donning scrub pants and shirt, placing a paper cap on my head and covers over my shoes, I felt a separation from the ordinary as I prepared to witness something remarkable. Yet I knew nothing and was simply an observer in this exclusive world of the operating room.

We entered the inner hallways leading to the operating rooms. Everything appeared to be in its proper place. Equipment was stored along the walls. Gurneys could be seen outside the various operating rooms where procedures were under way. I could peer through the glass windows to each room. I had no idea what was going on behind those doors, but it was unbelievably cool. There was the surgeon, standing and looking intently into a small space on a body covered in green cloth sheets. The bright lights hanging from the ceiling focused on that space. The anesthesiologist could be seen behind some large monster of a machine that had bellows moving up and down. The cardiac monitors could be seen with the heart waveforms showing up and disappearing in a fluorescent green color, accompanied by their unique beeping sound. Nobody was talking, yet everyone seemed to know their place and what to do. Nurses could be seen slapping instruments into the hand of the surgeon. I was mesmerized by the silent world I glimpsed through a little glass window in a door.

I followed my father toward his assigned operating room. We put on our facemasks, after he instructed me how to do so. I was too scared to say a word. As we walked into the room, the individuals in place—the various nurses, the anesthesiologist, the circulating nurse (the one who would be non-sterile and able to walk into and out of the room during the procedure to obtain equipment), and others—all greeted him, almost in unison. He returned their hellos and went immediately to the patient lying on the table. I recall seeing him take the patient's hand into his own and give it a gentle squeeze. The patient's tight, stressful facial expression seemed to melt into a broad smile—one of relief knowing that the Doctor, the champion, was present to offer protection and help. He would eliminate the medical problem. I remember being so proud of him at that moment. His very presence brought calm to the patient. He said little, yet at that moment he did so much to change the mood of the room.

After the introductions, the anesthesiologist proceeded to give an injection into the intravenous line in the patient's arm. I remember

CHAPTER 1 | *The Illness of Medicine*

watching the patient drift away and wondering whether that stuff would work on me in the same manner. As the anesthesiologist then intubated the patient—that is, placed a breathing tube into the patient's trachea to allow the anesthesiologist to control the patient's breathing—I recall clearly what my father did next. It has been impressed on my memory all these years, and I can see it as though he did it just yesterday.

With everyone going about their business—positioning the patient, moving equipment around, reviewing checklists, counting instruments—my father quietly went into the corner and sat down. He appeared to be in his own world, if for just a few moments. He was not engaged in any of the activity in the room. He seemed tranquil, almost meditative, and stared without expression, at nothing in particular. He sat in this position for about thirty seconds, and then he got up quickly and looked around to assess the status of things. He had returned from where he had been, and was engaged once more with the rest of the world. It was as if nothing had happened, minus those thirty seconds. He then asked me to come outside the room with him as he scrubbed his hands. Where had he gone and what had he thought about during that time-out? I wondered about it only briefly at the time. I would understand the answer to that question years later in my own life, but at that moment, I needed to get my own attention back into all that was going on. I was about to witness surgery!

What I observed was absolutely fascinating. I watched my dad operate on a child who suffered from being cross-eyed. The medical term is *strabismus*, which is a visual problem in which the eyes are not aligned properly. Consequently, the patient's eyes may look in different directions. By operating on the small muscles on the outside of the eyeball, or by moving the attachment point of the muscle on the eye, my father affected the eye's movement. I watched with fascination as the person I'd seen the night before using a hammer and a saw to construct basement cabinetry was now using those same hands to operate on an eye muscle that was possibly an eighth of an inch in width. His instruments were like a jeweler's; the suture material the width of a hair. I don't know if I took a single breath throughout the entire operation. It was mesmerizing, yet at the same time frightening. I witnessed a process I wasn't sure we were ever really supposed to see.

Leaving the hospital after my father had discussed his procedure with the family and had issued whatever postoperative instructions to the hospital staff, I remember being so proud to be his son. He'd performed his task with such humbleness about him; a man doing what he did for all the right reasons. I knew then and there that I wanted to be a surgeon one day. I wanted to be just like him.

CHAPTER 2

Medical School

So, what's it like to be a surgeon? I think that question has various answers on various levels. On the most primitive level, the fascination with peering inside ourselves, the better to understand how our bodies work, is almost as old as mankind itself. The understanding of *why* we work the way we do takes us into realms of human behavior best addressed by sociology, psychology, and cultural anthropology. So I'll keep it relatively simple and focus on the mechanics.

To open up and reach inside another human being is both fascinating and humbling, thrilling and frightening. It is unlike any other experience in life.

I remember my first days in anatomy lab as a freshman in medical school. Somehow biochemistry and physiology, though as critical as any other basic branches of medical knowledge, just didn't engage me the way anatomy did. Perhaps I needed a more concrete subject to study, one that didn't change with acidity or temperature, one that wasn't directly affected by the levels of oxygen or glucose—something I could see and feel. To actually open up a cadaver's

CHAPTER 2 | The Illness of Medicine

chest and look inside at the heart was glorious. Yet at the same time, it felt as though some of the mystery of life were being taken away. Then again, with each level of dissection, a *new* source of intrigue and awe was found. To put each discovery in context, however, meant realizing that anatomists have been identifying the same structures since the very first dissection. This was merely my turn, my chance to look inside.

Not nearly as interesting as the study of anatomy was the study of my fellow cadaver-sharing colleagues. Cadavers are expensive. As a consequence, medical students work on their "body" in groups. Typically, four students share a cadaver. Each member of the group participates in a relatively organized manner to complete the dissection of the various organ systems. My group of four young scientists included another male, who was the alpha among alphas, and two women who appeared to care little about what we were doing and who both went into a much more cerebral aspect of medicine: psychiatry. The alpha male was a sight to behold. I remember the very first day we had to bring in our new instruments. I brought in a scalpel, scissors, tweezers, and a few oddly shaped tools for probing. He brought with him an array of instruments so vast it could have been used for advanced neurosurgery. Apparently he had been a surgical orderly at some stage of life and had pilfered as many instruments as possible. No less than a hundred surgical tools were unloaded from his wheeled-in suitcase. I didn't know what most of them were for. He clearly thought he was going to be the next best thing in surgery (at this stage of learning, a medical student needs nothing more than a scalpel, scissors, and tweezers).

Michael J. Young, M.D.

As a consequence of having the next rising star in surgery in our group, managing the division of labor was going to be as tricky as was the dissection planned for each lab session.

The dissection of our cadaver began with the human hand. This was straightforward. The thing had a top and a bottom, and everything worked in a sensible manner—muscles pulled on tendons, which were attached to bones, which consequently moved as they were tugged on. The mechanical precision of the hand is unbelievably complex and yet so elegant in design and function. The absolute perfection of evolutionary development in it was jaw-dropping to me, and I wasn't even an engineer, just an observer of nature.

And so it started. We worked our way up the arm and into the shoulder. As we studied the different structures, each with its own flair and interest, I became more motivated. Every week I vowed to specialize in whatever anatomical structure we were currently working on. Each was inevitably more fascinating than the one before it.

My male cadaver-dissecting partner became increasingly obnoxious. I think he felt that an ability to dissect a cadaver meant he would have a unique ability to operate on living patients down the road. He was wrong on so many counts. A monkey can be taught where to cut. To develop the judgment on what *not* to cut is the key. To know when *not* to operate is what separates the superb surgeon from the ordinary one. That judgment is certainly not learned while dissecting a cadaver—nor, do I believe, is it easily learned while tending to living patients. A surgeon can master the techniques,

CHAPTER 2 | *The Illness of Medicine*

but the judgment of when to apply them is something a surgeon generally possesses or doesn't.

It was around the time of the shoulder dissection that I thought I would become a hand surgeon one day. Such work is a subspecialty of orthopedic and plastic surgery, involving a mixture of bone, muscle, tendon, blood vessels, and nerves. But then we entered the abdomen.

For reasons I still don't quite understand, the anatomy of the abdomen just didn't excite me as much as I had anticipated. It was fascinating, of course, but I had a hard time visualizing in three dimensions where things were going and whence they were coming. The upper extremity, with its obvious layers and direction of movement, made more sense to me. In the abdomen, by contrast, we now had a front and back (anterior and posterior), two sides, and everything in between. Organs were tucked into every available space, their own configuration affected not only by what was surrounding them but also by how the surrounding systems themselves matured and developed. The large liver, spleen, intestines, kidneys, were so individually complex not only in function but in form as well. Unlike bones and muscles, these structures seemed unique for each patient. Of course, gross similarities were obvious. But the dissection of each kidney, to this day, involves the recognition of slight variations in location and size, not only of the organ itself but of its constituent parts. For example, the entry and exit site for blood vessels to the same organ in different individuals can vary significantly. How each structure relates to its neighboring organs can potentially vary from patient to patient and can therefore dictate a surgical approach unique to each patient.

After the abdomen, we entered the pelvis. What a nightmare of structures. Now we had to deal with the three-dimensional, bowl-shaped pelvis and the plethora of nerves and vessels running therein. It was a struggle to assess which part of the tangle of nerves was coming and which was going, and to which organs. Many nerves were outbound while others were making their way up from the lower extremity. The complexity of it required as much imagination as understanding. To me, it was just a mass of confusion.

Now, too, we had the additional layer of gender-specific organs. In the female, the uterus, the ovaries, and their supporting structures. In the male, the prostate, the seminal vesicles, the vas deferens. I was lost, yearning to study the hand and arm again. The hand was flat and had a defined structure I could understand.

I clearly remember thinking to myself that I just had to get through this part of the anatomy, and then I'd never have to deal with it again. Memorize it, figure it out somehow, take the exam, and then just move on. But perhaps because the pelvic anatomy was so challenging for me, I ended up specializing in it. By forcing myself to learn it, possibly overlearn it, I eventually and truly came to appreciate it.

Moving on—thankfully for me at the time—we then entered the chest. As noted previously, opening the human chest induces a remarkable emotional reaction. It's not as though the heart actually controls any of our actions or reactions—quite the opposite, actually.

CHAPTER 2 | *The Illness of Medicine*

It reacts to everything else. But we have long associated the heart with all of our feelings, both good and bad. The connotation of the aching or joyous heart can be translated easily into every language. The heart is the perceived source for nearly all of our emotionally driven behavior. Upon opening the chest cavity, the excitement within my small group of cadaver explorers was palpable. Each of us peered intently into the open space as the heart came into view.

I felt a bit let down. After having heard possibly thousands of songs in my life describing how one's heart "felt," after having seen countless plays, operas, musicals, and movies all predicated on where people's hearts have "led them," I found the contents of our cadaver's chest cavity inconsistent with all that sentiment. I saw a slightly reddish gray muscle surrounded by a lot of fat tissue. It was just sitting there between the pinkish lungs. It wasn't moving. No music started playing, not even in my mind. No flashes of light or bells were going off. I'd half-expected to hear Julie Andrews start to sing from *The Sound of Music*. But the hills were not alive. After the four of us looked in, looked up at one another, and looked back in, I realized my disappointment was shared by the others. But nobody said a word. I felt a group sigh, and then we dutifully plodded on with our dissection.

We opened up the heart, just a massive muscle, one that works ceaselessly every second of every day. It's an absolute marvel of both form and function. But a thing of beauty to look at? Well, save it for the songs and operas.

Our next adventure was the dissection of the head and neck, the crossroads between our brain and body. The complexity of structure—going to or coming from somewhere else—was absolutely fascinating. Evolution had perfected this region of muscles, blood vessels, and nerves. I didn't need to be an engineer to appreciate the exquisite design and function. It was about at this time in my education that I also considered going into otolaryngology (ear, nose, and throat) as a specialty. The anatomy was just remarkable.

Our final area of study was the brain. The faculty had scheduled the neuroscience lectures to coordinate with our anatomy labs. It was mandatory for an understanding of what we were now studying. Yet with all the coordination and planning, a full understanding of the functioning of the human brain could never be accomplished in one, two, or even a hundred years' worth of classes. The brain is just that complex. Sure, mastering an understanding of bone or muscle or even such organs as the kidneys or liver requires a lifetime of devoted research, by which we can come to know at various basic levels how these structures work. But as we study the brain, so much of its basic function remains a great mystery. A black box. The myriad connections, the absolute volume of instructions and bodily functions being initiated by this organ, every second, makes the functioning of our largest, most complex computers appear to be comparatively simplistic.

And so, with the study of the various organ systems, each seemingly more complicated than the other, the decision of what actually to practice in medicine became less and less clear. It was all fascinating. It was all so difficult, even though I was learning about each of these topics at only a very superficial level—that of a first-

CHAPTER 2 | *The Illness of Medicine*

year medical student. Scientific lives over hundreds of years had been dedicated to trying to unravel the basic foundation of these organ systems and how they work.

Our second year of medical school was spent learning how things went wrong (pathology, pathophysiology), how to treat things when they did go wrong (for example, pharmacology) and finally how to examine whether things have gone wrong (the art of physical diagnosis). I didn't feel as though I were becoming a true scientist—someone who studies at the molecular and cellular levels how life works—but I was becoming a doctor, someone who understands the vocabulary of illness and who applies basic science to make the life of a patient better when something in the system has broken down.

Given my ability for visualization and my interest since childhood in taking things apart and then trying to put them back together, I knew becoming a surgeon was what I wanted to do. It's what I grew up with. It's what I saw from my father. I wanted to be part of that world.

CHAPTER 3

Residency

As far back as the age of about eleven, I knew I wanted to be a doctor. Prior to that I thought I was destined to be a veterinarian. My father and mother joked with me during my youth that I could always dig ditches for a living, as long as I received my M.D. first. And so, it was decided.

My father, of course, was a physician, as had been my grandfather and great-grandfather. The reasons for my going into medicine were clear: I wanted to be like my dad. As previously discussed, he was an ophthalmologist. But what he actually did for a living was less important to me than the manner in which he did it. He was a kind, gentle person, and I had always looked up to him. He was respected by everyone I knew, and his interest in understanding how things work rubbed off on me. He always wanted to build things, to fix them, to make them better. This encouraged my interest in science, and since I also had two older brothers who were either in medical training or on that same trajectory, it seemed the right thing for me to do as well. If nothing else, I wanted to be able to understand and participate in the dinnertime conversation.

CHAPTER 3 | The Illness of Medicine

I entered college with one intent: to go to medical school. I remember my dormitory friends constantly reminding me of how low the acceptance rate was for applicants to medical school. I was undeterred by their pessimism. In fact, it only fortified my resolve. I studied hard and was academically successful as a student. I achieved my goal and was accepted to the medical school of my choice.

Then I learned that medical school was a unique experience—beyond anything undergraduate accomplishment had prepared me for. The work load alone far exceeded that of even my hardest semesters in college. Medical education is divided essentially into two segments. During the preclinical years, the student is pounded with physiology, anatomy, pharmacology, microbiology, and biochemistry. Then two years are spent on clinical rotations, during which the student learns the basics of being a doctor. Rotations involve the student spending hands-on time with practitioners in various fields of medicine, including, for example, general surgery, internal medicine, pediatrics, and psychiatry. The last year of medical school is spent learning the subspecialties, such as orthopedics, otolaryngology, plastic surgery, and urology. It is during rotations that the student is faced with the daunting task of deciding which branch of medicine he or she desires eventually to pursue.

Although the romantic ideal is to practice in an area of medicine for which one seems to have a calling, the reality of choosing a field is much more difficult. As with medical school itself, the number of those applying for residency far exceeds the number of those accepted. (*Residency* refers to the period of dedicated specialty training following graduation from medical school, and involves the medical field one intends to pursue as a career). The difference, of course, is that at this point all of the applicants have successfully cleared the previous hurdles. They are all highly accomplished people seeking to continue their missions.

While selecting a field of interest, it is equally important to recognize that the branch of medicine one pursues will determine far more than just how one spends one's days treating disease. It will determine how one sleeps and eats, the hours one works, the length and quality of time one spends at home. The chosen field of study will also determine the newly minted doctor's friends and what opportunities he or she has to develop other aspects of life. The general surgeon is up at dawn and is often the last physician to leave the hospital. By comparison, the dermatologist rarely, if ever, has to deal with emergencies. Many dermatologists don't even carry a pager.

I decided to practice urology and looking back, it was an excellent choice. Urologists are confronted with few true emergencies, have myriad procedures and technological tools at their disposal, and enjoy a broad mix of both office and hospital exposure. It is one of those fields popular with medical students interested in a surgical career.

The process of entering residency has undergone changes over the years. In the past, upon completion of medical school, if one

CHAPTER 3 | *The Illness of Medicine*

wanted additional training, the student would apply to various well-known programs or contact potential mentors throughout the country and interview for an open position. Selecting a program was difficult. Where one trained would have a direct influence on the people the resident would meet, and this could subsequently determine the people with whom or for whom one would work upon completing residency. (As an aside, given that graduates of medical school are generally in their mid-twenties, their opportunities for meeting a significant other—assuming they haven't already—are affected by the type of program they choose, the work and study hours involved, and the location of the training.) Thirty years ago, if an applicant and a mentor met and got along, the mentor placed some phone calls and reached out to the medical-school counselors and the residency program director to discuss the applicant. An agreement for training was a bond between teacher and apprentice.

In urology, starting around 1990, the residency match program was initiated. As its name implies, the program was designed to match the applicant to a residency program, but it was also a means of making the process of application and acceptance more equitable. No longer was a referral from a well-placed medical-school instructor or friend to the director of the desired program the main requisite for acceptance into the program. The process was highly organized and fair. On their applications, the students ranked programs according to their preference. The program directors did the same for the applicants they interviewed. A computer program would match the two, weighting things toward the students' choices to the extent possible during the matching process.

Michael J. Young, M.D.

I matched to my first-choice program and then began the long process of becoming a urologist. This mandated completing two years of general surgery, followed by four years of urology residency. The first year of residency, also known as an internship, primarily involves being the scut dog for everyone else above you. You're the first one called for nearly every problem that occurs during the day or night. Whether one has the ability, understanding, or maturity to recognize the true nature of each problem varies among interns—and situations. It's a difficult time. In my experience, one's year was divided between actually being on the general surgery service, managing inpatient and outpatient surgical issues (hernias, gallbladders, intestinal surgical conditions, etc.), and spending time on various surgical subspecialties (vascular, cardiothoracic, orthopedic, plastic surgery, etc.). The intern spent very little time actually learning or performing surgery. The job was to observe, handle the hour-to-hour postoperative problems, and basically be responsible for knowing each patient's every nuance. There was little rest. There was no sympathy and very little empathy from the more senior residents or staff regarding what was going on in your life: personal or professional. Unlike today, there were no work-hour limits, and there was no relief for being ill or exhausted. It was a miserable time in my life—probably the hardest of my training—but also the year I learned the most about myself, as I gained exposure to a mountain of medical conditions and took responsibility for and resolved various problems. When I was a surgical intern, general surgery was looked upon as the "balls" of the hospital. I suspect it had earned that reputation long before

CHAPTER 3 | The Illness of Medicine

my experience. General surgeons were the first to be called for any patient that needed interventional treatment. And, yes, in practical terms, that meant the intern was expected to be the first of that service to respond when the help call was placed.

The second year of residency is an inch above internship. You're still of lowly status, and the shit still runs downhill, but at least you have that intern to exploit when necessary. I found the second year to be one of increased responsibility, and as I was now the in-house backup for the intern, it was significantly more difficult emotionally.

I think the hardest experience a young physician ever has to deal with, and one that is never forgotten, is the first patient death for which he or she feels accountable.

I can take myself back to that time as though it were yesterday. I have played out the events so many times in my head that the sounds, the anxiety I felt, even the smells of the chaotic activity surrounding my patient's demise, are just a thought away.

I was the surgical resident on call for the Veterans Administration (VA) hospital on an absolutely perfect Saturday in August. Although my residency program was at a university setting, we spent time training (rotating) at a nearby VA hospital. As the second-year resident, I had the responsibility of covering the surgical intensive care unit (SICU), which housed some of the sickest patients in the hospital. All had undergone at least one or more complicated surgical procedure. Many were not doing well.

Michael J. Young, M.D.

One of the patients I was assigned to cover was in his mid-sixties, recovering from open-heart surgery three days prior. I had learned this was a redo cardiac bypass, meaning he had had open-heart surgery previously and the vessels that had formed the bypass that is, the blood vessels that had been removed from the legs and then attached before and after the native, obstructed vessels of the heart had also become occluded. This meant he had had his chest opened for heart surgery a second time in his life. He was also a brittle diabetic, and obese, and had an additional history of COPD (chronic obstructive pulmonary disease) related to his ongoing habit of smoking three packs of cigarettes a day. Not a healthy patient. Certainly, things have changed in the thirty years since I was a second-year surgical resident covering the SICU. Hospital coverage is significantly more regulated, and the cell phone now exists. At that time, however, I was the physician responsible for his care and management. There was no senior surgical resident, fellow, or attending physician in the hospital that perfect Saturday.

I remember I came to work early and drove in with the windows down, trying to take in as much fresh air as I could, knowing that I would be in the hospital for the next twenty-four hours without any break. I also knew the VA would be stifling that day as the air-conditioning was basically nonexistent and the on-call sleeping rooms were up on the ninth floor without any windows. That wonderful morning air would become oppressive in the old, poorly ventilated building. It was going to be a hot one.

I made rounds with the fellow upon my arrival. A fellow is a physician who, after completing medical school and residency,

CHAPTER 3 | The Illness of Medicine

is obtaining additional subspecialty training. In this case, I was with the cardiothoracic fellow, seeing his patients in the SICU. All seemed fine. There were three patients on ventilators—breathing machines for those who are too ill or weak, or still too heavily sedated after recent surgery, to breathe on their own. The SICU had a smattering of other postoperative patients, many of whom could have been discharged to a standard surgical floor. It was the weekend, however, and their doctors had elected to keep them in the SICU for good measure (no worry or even a moment's thought about the additional insurance costs that extra SICU days at the VA would entail). And then there was our patient, recovering from his redo bypass procedure. He looked okay. He had been extubated (the breathing tube from the ventilator had been removed), and he was breathing on his own. Slightly labored breathing was noted, but he stated that he felt fine, and his blood oxygenation saturation levels (O2 sats) were acceptable. These measurements were made from a monitor (a pulse oximeter) placed on the patient's finger.

Having completed his rounds, the fellow left for home, and I was responsible to watch over the patients. It's never a good feeling to be alone in a hospital, on a weekend, without close backup, particularly with only one solid year of surgical residency (internship) under one's belt. Actually, it was scary as hell—a feeling of constant anxiety mixed with occasional panic right down to the gut. But hey, I was a surgeon, and I knew experience would gradually overtake the anxiety, one day. I just didn't have a clue when that one day was going to happen.

Michael J. Young, M.D.

I was a rather compulsive resident. (I became a rather compulsive surgical attending years later.) I must have checked on my patient's clinical status ten times that day. Perhaps that was part of the problem. I think that if you look at the same situation over and over in a relatively brief time frame, you become less aware of the subtle changes. If you observe the same situation over a longer time interval, changes become more obvious. Any serious medical situation mandates not only repeated assessment but also knowing at what interval to repeat the assessment. Getting a chest x-ray every hour on a patient with pneumonia makes no sense. Get it taken every twenty-four hours, and then one can see important changes.

I suspect that in observing my patient so often, even sitting at his bedside for long stretches, I was failing to note slow changes in his respiratory effort. His pulse oximeter indicated that he was maintaining a reasonable level of blood oxygenation—reasonable, that is, for a patient who could not expand his lungs completely due to the recent surgery in his chest and also due to his underlying respiratory disease (COPD). But what was changing, subtly, was his effort and the amount of energy being expended by him to maintain that steady oxygenation. As the day progressed, his O2 saturations were slowly diminishing. He continued to express to me that he was "fine." Until suddenly, he wasn't.

Around eleven o'clock at night, I became alarmed by his breathing. He was really working hard to get air in and out. His O2 sats were acceptable, but not great. They were going down slowly. What I failed to realize—what I did not have enough experience to realize

CHAPTER 3 | The Illness of Medicine

at the time—was that his breathing efforts were not sustainable. He was losing the battle to breathe, it just hadn't happened yet. I wondered if he was fluid overloaded, and if this was preventing his lungs from being able to appropriately oxygenate the blood. Was he having pain? Was there a blood clot to his lungs (pulmonary embolism)? Was his heart, which had recently been operated on, getting constricted by a fluid buildup at the surgical site? I didn't know the answer to these questions that were racing through my head. But I did know that I had an urgent problem in front of me as he suddenly appeared more ashen in color. His O2 saturations dropped precipitously, and he started to lose consciousness.

I cursed myself for failing to anticipate this outcome and called a code blue, an alarm for a cardiac/respiratory arrest. As a surgical intern, I had been to many codes. It was the surgical intern's job to be present and available to obtain a central line—that is, vascular access for fluids, drugs, and monitoring in these situations. I had witnessed and been trained in the procedures for advanced CPR. But this was different from all the other codes I had been part of. This was *my* patient. I'd watched him so carefully throughout the day, but I'd failed to observe the subtle changes, until they hit a critical threshold of respiratory failure.

He stopped breathing. I ran to the head of the bed and tried to intubate him—to place the breathing tube into his trachea so that we could attach him to the ventilator and take over his breathing for him. I couldn't get the damn tube in. He was still semiconscious, and he bit down reflexively on my hand as I tried to pry open his mouth and place the half-inch-wide tube down his throat and into his trachea. My hand was now bleeding into his mouth, and he was turning blue. I could hear the code-blue alarms going off in the background. People were rushing in to help. But I was at his head, he was my patient, and I knew I was losing him. Everything became a blur. People were shouting orders, my hand was stinging from the bite, and the noise in my head became overwhelming.

Finally, as he lost consciousness, I was able to slip the endotracheal tube past his vocal cords and into his trachea. We connected him to the ventilator, and we stabilized his vital signs. His body had survived the arrest.

Unfortunately, his brain had not.

He never regained consciousness. In fact, for weeks we observed him in the intensive care unit. Once he was medically stable we moved him to a step-down unit. I saw him multiple times a day. His family was always at the bedside.

"How did this happen?" they would ask.

"Why did I not electively intubate him sooner?" I would ask myself.

Eventually, months after it was ascertained that the patient would not recover and that cognitive function was not evident, the family elected to disconnect him from life support. He died. A small part of me did as well.

It took me the rest of that second year of residency to realize that for all the training, the knowledge, and the voluminous reading and study that had gotten me to this point in my career, there was no

CHAPTER 3 | The Illness of Medicine

better teacher than experience. I learned. But I was also angry that the system had put me in that position—alone, on a weekend, just over a year after graduating medical school, without any immediate support or supervision. I would never forget that episode. Ever.

The following years were spent in my field of choice, and a fascinating field it is. Urology is the study of the genitourinary system, which comprises an extraordinarily complex set of organs that includes the kidneys; the ureters, which are the structures that connect the kidneys and the lower urinary tract (the bladder, prostate, and urethra); and, in the male, the external genitalia. Urology also encompasses the study of male fertility in reproduction.

Its area of potential surgical intervention encompasses the chest, the abdomen, and the pelvis. Along with covering a lot of real estate, it involves understanding the physiology and function of the systems within those structures, and their relationship to everything else in the body. The residency is long, and one studies the treatments encompassing everything from the most basic of procedures (circumcisions) to advanced cancer or reconstructive surgical cases.

Training continues over the years through observation of one's mentors and through constant study, with one's involvement in surgical procedures increasing as skill level and understanding mature. It is a slow process, given the volume of information residents must assimilate and the skills they must eventually master before going out on their own. The residency program must assure itself, its governing body (The American Board of Urology) and the public that the individual who labels himself a urologist, having been trained at an approved program, is indeed capable of managing both simple and complex urological conditions. The question that is of course unknown is whether that graduating urologist, after five-six years of training, has the judgment to know when, and if, to intervene.

Teaching someone how to sew is not difficult. Likewise, teaching a young surgeon to cut here and repair something else there is tedious, but achievable. Teaching that same young person the *judgment* to know whether to operate *is* difficult.

As a resident, one can feel empowered as one's stature within the program rises. I can remember being so impressed by my more senior residents' knowledge. But for all their knowledge and all their confidence, they were still residents. They made few significant management decisions on their own. They usually had an attending physician behind them, someone effectively watching their backs, always helping them navigate surgical difficulties.

Learning to understand one's limitations as a surgeon, as a physician with the responsibility to consider all options in caring for one's patient—including the option not to intervene—is, I believe, the hallmark of a surgical education. Certainly, a physician may *physically* treat his last patient similarly to his very first. Same procedure for the same problem. But the process of understanding the situation, the nuances that may differ consequentially between treating the first and last patient, defines the *experience* of practicing medicine that cannot be taught. It cannot be read in a book or gleaned

CHAPTER 3 | The Illness of Medicine

from articles in a journal. The experience of understanding medicine simply must be lived through, while making a considerable effort to learn and retain how each event and outcome transpired—both the good and the not so good. But always learn from the experience.

As I progressed to my sixth and final year of training, I found myself frequently reliving my encounter four years earlier as a second-year surgical resident, when I misinterpreted the warning signs of an impending respiratory arrest. Nothing anyone could have said in a lecture, or in books I could have read, would have prepared me for that series of events at that stage of my training. But I learned from that episode, and as I was going forward toward completing this phase of my medical education, I realized that many more difficult lessons were to come. I knew they were just around the corner, and would happen again and again. I could read, I could study, I could observe my professors. But ultimately, what I needed most was experience—again, the ultimate teacher in medical education.

Not that I didn't have outstanding teachers in real life as well. The chairman of the urology department was a tremendous role model—both an outstanding urologist and, more important, a kind and fair person. He pushed me to learn, to become better. Other attending physicians in the department were becoming friends and mentors of mine as well. One in particular had an extraordinary skill in surgery matched equally by his use of a knife in his kitchen. I am grateful to all my teachers for having the fortitude and patience to teach a batch of budding young surgeons year after year. It was only after I launched my private practice and began supervising residents on my own that I truly appreciated how difficult teaching the next generation can be. Those students are learning on your patients, while looking to you for answers and guidance. It is truly a daunting experience to hand a scalpel to someone and tell him what to do with it, but not half as daunting as it is to be the patient who lies on the table, giving you all of his trust.

When I went into my very first procedure after starting my private practice, I understood the meditative pause I'd watched my father observe that time I'd accompanied him into the operating room so many years before. It was his moment of reflection, of respect and self-awareness for what he was about to do. My father later told me that if you don't shake in your boots a bit before surgery, then you don't belong in the operating room. He was so very right.

My formal medical education phase was over. It was now time to practice medicine.

CHAPTER 4

How Things Have Changed

My, how things have changed in our attitude toward physicians. I recall what a big deal it was going to the pediatrician. I think I was informed well in advance of the appointment, certainly no less than a month out.

We had to wear our "nice" clothes—not the ones we played in, and not the ones we prayed in, but nice clothes. We took our baths or showers before our appointment. As much as I liked my pediatrician, I was still scared to go to his office. But I think the only doctor that I was absolutely terrified to see was the dentist. He never stopped drilling, even when I raised my hand high in the air, as instructed to do if in pain.

But visiting the pediatrician was different. He was a kind, gentle man, never in a rush. The waiting area had dark wood paneling. It was cheap, but it covered old walls. He had a large fish tank that all of the kids, including me, would stare into with awe, our noses pushed up to the glass. Are large fish tanks mandatory in a pediatrician's office? If not, they should be. A tank full of fish swimming in no particular pattern can keep a child amused for

CHAPTER 4 | *The Illness of Medicine*

a really long time. He had magazines that required interaction from the children. We had to find the objects hidden in the images. However, without fail, the word puzzles in those magazines were always halfway completed by another child. Coloring books and crayons were always strewn about the floor.

My pediatrician's receptionist/assistant/nurse (one person) always had a smile on her face. She peered out frequently from behind the hole cut in the wall between the waiting area and the front office. The typewriter could be heard clicking away in that uneven pattern of tic-tic—tictic. She was dressed in white, head to toe.

I waited quietly, but anxiously, to be summoned back into the examination room. I can remember the door to the receptionist's work area opening up and hearing my name announced. It's odd, but the waiting room was never full, and it was only maybe ten feet by twenty feet in size. Announcements probably weren't necessary. But what struck me most upon being called for my examination was that the waiting area was dark and the receptionist's work area was brightly lit. So when the door opened and the figure of the nurse was seen standing there, she was always backlit. I couldn't really see details, just the outline of a lady with a nurse's cap on. It wasn't until my mom and I would walk up in front of her that I could actually see her face.

I would follow her instructions diligently. I wanted to be a good patient. The exam room—it was always chilly. I was instructed to change into one of those gowns designed for a medical examination. Who designed these things? I remember trying to figure out which was the front and which the back. I never could tie it right.

Michael J. Young, M.D.

Eventually, I think I would just tie it whatever way the tie-strings were dangling on a given exam day. A thermometer was then stuck into my mouth, always just a bit too far for comfort. And then the nurse would leave. I couldn't talk, not with a thermometer placed somewhere next to my uvula. I was cold. And the darn exam gown was always tugging somewhere because I never put it on as the designer, who was obviously never a patient, intended. We waited. Although I was healthy and knew I needed nothing more than a routine inoculation, I was still scared. Maybe it was because my mom was anxious. She didn't fare well in doctors' offices.

The doctor walked in, paper chart in hand—something we don't see anymore. He would always shake my hand, and his hand was always damp. I assumed it was from his having just washed it after seeing his last patient. His hands were cold. Or maybe it was just because the room felt about fifty degrees. I would hop onto the exam table, where the roll paper over the vinyl table covering would stick to the back of my legs. The doctor would then calmly sit down, peer through his reading glasses, and look at my records. He wouldn't say a word. Then he would look up and start chatting with my mom about what seemed to be everything under the sun. There was no hurry in his approach. Both he and my mom respected one another. He was what a doctor was supposed to be: calm, confident. He had a plan. And he listened.

The exam would start by his placing the ice-cold stethoscope on my chest. He would move it around and have me breathe in and out. After about five of the largest breaths I could muster, I would start to feel a little dizzy. He would feel my "stomach." His cold hands

CHAPTER 4 | *The Illness of Medicine*

just never seemed to get any warmer. And then, after the doctor completed his exam, he would tell my mom and me, again in his gentle manner, that all was just fine. But one more thing, which he would leave to the end: I needed a shot.

What I learned from him, and what I subsequently applied to my own practice when I was on the other side of the table: never lie to the patient about how much something will hurt. It was time for my shot, and he told me, "This will hurt a bit." He never said this is like "a little bee sting," or some other idiotic expression that had no relevance to most seven-year-olds. How many kids actually know what a bee sting feels like? And bee stings, as I learned later in life, hurt like hell! He said it would hurt, plain and simple. So I braced myself, bit my lower lip, and endured my shot. When it was over, and slight tears welled up in my eyes, he would smile and pat me on the head. He'd kept his word, and done his job. To the end of my days practicing, I would do the same for my patients before my procedures on them (involving hypodermics or otherwise). Let them honestly know what to expect, and they will leave with respect both for you, their physician, and for themselves, for having withstood what they'd been told would be painful. Their trust will not be gained by misdirection and attempts at verbally minimizing the discomfort they are about to experience.

I would then get to select a sucker from the container on my way out—always an orange one—and off we went. I was relieved, satisfied, and now ready to tackle whatever came up, my confidence restored from a cold, damp hand, a shot, and a smile.

* * * * * * * * * *

Michael J. Young, M.D.

Fast-forward decades later. I would arrive at my office an hour before the patients were scheduled for their appointments. My first step was to boot up my computer and begin to review the onslaught of new "tasks"—reviewing lab results, pathology reports, and x-ray reports and, of course, returning patients' emails that had come in on the "electronic portal" to their medical records. I would make my list of who needed to be called and when. Throughout my practice, I made a habit of returning certain calls at only certain times of the day, and informed patients of results on only certain days of the week. For instance, I would never call a patient on Friday regarding a recent biopsy, unless the news was good. It just bothered me to ruin someone's weekend by informing him on Friday that he had a newly diagnosed prostate cancer. The cancer would still be there the following Monday, without any progression or change. On the other hand, good news, a negative biopsy, was never delayed. Those fortunate patients were always called as soon as I received the reports. The delivery of x-ray and lab results was similarly based on the urgency of the matter, the relevance to a condition, and how a particular patient would likely react. The *art of* medicine began with the basics: knowing how and when to inform a patient of his or her medical information.

Patients would arrive. I always prided myself on having relevant and contemporary magazines in the waiting room. Most of my patients were older men. We had golf and sporting magazines. We had investment magazines. I tried to make sure they were kept current. I can easily remember going to doctors' offices and seeing magazines that were so ancient I had to struggle to remember

CHAPTER 4 | The Illness of Medicine

what the headlines on the magazine covers were even referring to. Leafing through a stack of old magazines in a doctor's office and finding a *Sports Illustrated* with the winners of the Super Bowl from five years ago on the cover just does not promote confidence. You wonder what else in this office is also five years out of date.

But in this modern, technological era, we have become prisoners to our own attempts to improve understanding. No longer does a patient come to the office, hand in his or her insurance information, sign in, and sit down. Now we have endless pages of information we must solicit from the patients, related to everything from their current medical complaint to their lifestyle and even their psychological status. Are they happy or sad today? Seriously. Much of this is mandated by the insurance providers, who can't possibly think a busy orthopedic surgeon actually cares if a patient is feeling a bit melancholy today. More important, they can't honestly think the surgeon will read that crap. What the doctor wants to learn from the patient is where things hurt, and when.

Then let's move on to page twenty of the encounter form where details of one's insurance policy are listed. This is the point where most patients begin to sweat. Rarely does a patient clearly understand what is covered, and what isn't, by his or her insurance policy, or when a copay is necessary. The policy variations are limitless and numbing. And after filling out this encounter form, the patient is then to walk into the exam room, wait a half an hour, and then have blood pressure taken. "My, it's a little high today," the nurse or medical assistant might state in mock surprise. I wonder why it would be.

Michael J. Young, M.D.

But to cap it off, to make the "encounter experience" all the more uncomfortable, we have the marvels of the *electronic encounter form*. No longer does the patient have to sit cross-legged just to keep the twenty sheets of paper on his lap from falling everywhere. Now he can fill out his forms with the convenience of a tablet computer. My elderly patients, who had so proudly driven themselves to my office, found parking, climbed stairs, and negotiated their way to their doctor's reception area, were now confronted with this perplexity, this dubious convenience. The fonts were often too small, making reading the fine print even more difficult. Also, it's bad enough peppering with questions those patients who are coming in for a medical problem and who might be scared of a new diagnosis of cancer, but it's bordering on cruel to compel them to answer by way of a newfangled device whose interface baffles them. Often my office staff would need to assist, or even complete the forms for the patients. This would not only back up the office flow but would also add to staff frustration at not being able to get other work done. So now the anxious patient is more agitated, the office flow is being delayed at the gates, and the office staff is overworked. And let's not forget the last pearl of joy in this experience:

The referral is missing or outdated. Sound the alarms! Prepare for battle stations!

What a mess.

The patient who has come for help, who is worried about his condition, who is late because of traffic, and who has completed his encyclopedia-like forms on a tablet he could barely read is now told

CHAPTER 4 | The Illness of Medicine

that his referral is a) missing, b) expired, or c) not applicable to his current appointment issue. This meant an explosion was about to occur in my front office. And it did so with regularity.

So what is this referral nonsense anyway? The referral system came about as a means of limiting unnecessary consultations with specialists, of more closely tracking the health care a patient receives, and—just as important to the managed-care providers—of more closely tracking the *performance* of health care *practitioners* for the scrutiny of their administrators. For patients in an HMO (health maintenance organization), the referral is the piece of paper, obtainable from their primary care physician, that allows them to consult a specialist. It represents an imposing attempt to manage and regulate health care by preventing excessive interventions, surgeries, imaging, and lab testing. From my perspective, as a doctor, it was worthless. To the HMO managers and administrators, it is a priceless form of leverage. No patient in their plan can get anything done without first acquiring this official piece of paper.

So the primary care physician performs testing that suggests the possibility of, say, prostate cancer. There is concern, and the patient is now referred to me, the specialist, for continued evaluation. The referral lets me know that I have the permission to see the patient and that I will be paid for this evaluation according to a prearranged fee schedule. If I actually saw the patient and made the diagnosis without his first proffering and my first verifying the holy paper, then I risked being denied payment and the patient risked having any treatment thereafter (related to the current condition) denied by the insurer/HMO. Hence the anxiety of all involved over referrals. Yet the odd thing is that nearly every referral initiated by a primary care physician is granted by the insurer/HMO, meaning the attempt at limiting excessive intervention, testing, imaging, etc., has come to naught. So what is the purpose of the referral process—other than to track the system? There probably isn't one. But don't bother taking time off from work to show up for your x-ray or lab test, or to drive a hundred miles to see the specialist, without that damn referral form.

Yet my elderly new patient didn't bring his referral. Possibly he didn't understand how important it was to do so. Perhaps the importance of the document was not made sufficiently clear to him at his primary physician's office. My patient must now sit down and wait. My already overburdened office staff must take yet more time and contact the referring provider to obtain the necessary approval. It doesn't matter that we had previously called the patient and informed him of the need to bring the paper. It doesn't matter that the patient was informed of the central importance of the referral when he obtained his insurance, or that he probably was recently reminded of this importance at his primary care physician's office. The guy doesn't have it, and he's in my waiting area. Patients keep coming through the door. Someone now needs help with the computer tablet, and she doesn't speak English. My receptionist is about to have a meltdown, and for good reason. I really miss the days of my pediatrician. Maybe I need to get a fish tank too, one for the waiting room and one for my private office. Watching the fish swim back and forth does calm the nerves a bit, doesn't it?

CHAPTER 4 | *The Illness of Medicine*

Finally ... the referral gets faxed. The primary care physician was out of the office, so additional delays occurred, but all is now in order. Fine. That was easy.

My new patient comes back into the exam room. He is seen by one of my medical assistants, who will take vital signs (temperature, blood pressure, pulse, respiratory rate) and record the patient's height and weight. The assistant, too, will need to update her own computer record of the patient's profile—pertaining to changes in medications or other personal information. By the time I walk into the room, the patient is either so exhausted from the intake process that he is like a lamb, or so wired-up and angry at the process that apologies and reassurances are necessary.

"Now what are you here for today?" I ask. And finally, we begin.

A FEW OBSERVATIONS

Having witnessed the "patient intake process" perhaps a hundred or so times per week, for years, I came away with several interesting observations.

For instance, younger patients had a consistently different attire than did older patients. My older patients would still "get dressed" for the doctor, wearing nice clothes—even a tie on the retired eighty-year-olds. The younger patients (men presenting, say, for a vasectomy or women for evaluation of recurrent urinary tract infections) were frequently in jeans, shorts, or tank tops. Over time I also learned that the severity of a medical issue often directly correlated with how patients dressed for the appointment. A concerned patient with a more serious condition would dress for the part.

I also noted a difference in who accompanied the patient. Heterosexual males and females would typically come into the exam room alone. Gay patients, male or female, nearly always came in with their partners. Transgender patients varied. I don't know if this was a matter of trust in and dependency on the partner, or of the partner's need to simultaneously evaluate the physician. But I could almost always accurately assess sexual orientation before I even said "hello." Most examinations were uneventful. The majority of office appointments were postoperative assessments involving various stages of recovery, simply to make sure all was well. Cancer patients without evidence of progression were always a pleasure to see. To hear what they were doing with their lives now that the cancer treatment was over was always worth hearing. I admired them for what they had gone through, and how they had dealt with their diagnosis. I suspected that some of my colleagues, given their arrogance and lack of sensitivity, would not have fared as well had they been the ones undergoing diagnosis and treatment.

I found that most of my fellow physicians were caring, concerned, and dedicated to their patient needs. Others, however, some with whom I worked quite closely, changed over the years. They ceased being the "concerned physician." They became obsessed with making money and comparing their status among their "physician friends," that status often measured in metrics that had nothing to do with why they initially went into medicine. Or maybe it did.

CHAPTER 4 | *The Illness of Medicine*

Sometimes, I guess, it just takes some time for a person's true motivation to show itself.

The more difficult appointments were the post-biopsy cancer discussions, which—even when done well—were never easy. Such appointments needed to be tailored to the patient's understanding of the problem and to how quickly the patient could assimilate the information that needed to be reviewed.

I learned that most patients remembered very little of what was said after the word *cancer*. I always insisted that patients with a cancer diagnosis come to the office with someone else. This additional person had more objective ears and could later help the patient refer back to forgotten parts of the discussion. We would meet a second time, usually a couple of weeks later. I wanted the patient to have an opportunity to read what I had given him or her, to mull things over, and to formulate questions.

This process took time. Knowing how much time depended upon my individual assessment of the patient. I found two extreme types of reactions always a bit curious, and also troubling to deal with.

On the one hand, there were the patients who assumed no responsibility for treatment, and would delegate this entirely to the doctor. "Whatever you say, Doc." This was never good, and rarely led to the desired outcome without significant bumps along the way. Such a patient would always claim ignorance and never actively participate in any decision-making, instead simply going along with the treatment. However, when problems occurred or unexpected events happened, the patient would immediately claim that nobody had told him anything. The other difficult patient type was the overly suspicious individual. He wanted records of everything. He brought in reams of printed material from the internet, and he always had a family member somewhere on the planet who was "an expert" in their field. It didn't mean an expert in urology, but an expert nonetheless and therefore a valid reference point for the patient. These patients were difficult, not because of their medical condition. More than likely I knew how they would fare and what needed to be done from the time we began the discussion. Rather, they were difficult because everything for them, with them, around them, was a challenge. Making decisions was a challenge for them, as was dealing with problems. Progress was slow and tedious, as this type of patient had literally too much information to process and rarely delegated decision-making to anyone. Deciding what and where to eat for dinner was probably even an arduous task for this personality type.

One of the more onerous tasks in the office is having to schedule a patient for surgery. After a meeting with the patient in which the problem has been identified, the doctor discusses and reviews options for managing the problem. This may necessitate several more appointments, with imaging, lab studies, and outside consultation. Often, matters are then reviewed once more with the patient's family or partner. The next step is to find a date. This mandates a dance of sorts, to find when both the doctor's schedule and the patient's schedule (what with work, home care, transportation, recovery period, and other family considerations) are open or can be cleared. After a general time frame has been

CHAPTER 4 | *The Illness of Medicine*

agreed upon, the final variable is the availability of the operating room. The OR in each facility has its own set of time constraints and protocols.

Surgery can be performed at any number of locations, and the decision on where to have it performed is predicated on a number of issues. Doctor and patient must decide on the degree of intervention necessary. Obviously, procedures requiring simple local anesthetic (meaning that no general anesthesia is necessary, and that the surgical site will be numbed with a "local" injection) can be performed just about anywhere—in the office, at an outpatient surgical center, or, of course, in a hospital. Whether to rely on local anesthesia is dictated by the patient's pain tolerance and desire for expedience (local is always quicker than general anesthesia) as well as by the surgeon's preference. There are patients who would prefer to have most anything done in the office, to minimize costs and time. Others are more squeamish, or have poor pain tolerance, and want everything performed under general anesthesia. During my time, I saw the entire gamut of reactions to procedures. How patients fared, I found, had less to do with the actual physical discomfort of an intervention than with their anticipation/perception of the procedure.

For example, I performed vasectomies (tying off the vas deferens, the tube that carries sperm to the outside world) regularly in the office. My technique never varied in over twenty years—same procedure, same incisions, same anesthetic. I had patients who got so anxious they literally passed out. This occurred in some patients as I was merely beginning to clean the area of the procedure, prior to any manipulation or incision. On the other end of the spectrum, I once performed a vasectomy on a former Green Beret. He informed me that pain was "not in his vocabulary," so he did not want to have any anesthetic—at all. Okay. I performed the procedure without anesthesia, and I'm not sure he even blinked while it was happening. Afterward, he got up off the table, said "thank you," and went on his way.

* * * * * * * * * *

So, we have a patient who needs a procedure. Assuming the patient requires general anesthesia, the next decision is whether or not this can be done in an outpatient surgical center or must be done in the hospital. Often, the surgical center—which typically specializes in performing a high volume of a narrow range of procedures—is less expensive and more efficient than a large hospital. Hospitals were initially designed for inpatient care. As they have tried to transform into faster outpatient-type facilities, they still seem to be hindered by bulk and size. Processes are slower. The check-in, check-out mechanism is cumbersome. The operating rooms in hospitals generally perform larger cases, so delays are frequent, and this makes it more difficult to estimate the time requirements for each case. Emergencies can come in at any time, causing a backup of scheduled procedures. Often the surgery departments are complex and can be quite large. Multiple individuals are involved in the scheduling process. Again, these are all reasons why hospitals

CHAPTER 4 | The Illness of Medicine

generally have a difficult time competing with surgical centers, which are significantly smaller, more efficient, and consequently more convenient (for physician and patient) for many minor surgical procedures.

In many cases, the decision of where to have the general-anesthetic procedure is determined by the surgical needs. Hospital operating rooms are well equipped, and if a particular instrument requested by the surgeon isn't on hand, hospitals are able to procure it prior to the surgery date. Also influencing the decision: what is safest for the patient in terms of anesthetic needs, anticipated blood loss, and possible complications? What type of physical issues does the patient have—both in terms of the problem being repaired and in his overall health? What are the postoperative requirements for a stable, smooth recovery? The potential need for postoperative nursing care, pain management, various levels of monitoring, etc., must be taken into account. Again, we must err on the side of caution. The procedure needs to be performed where all of these issues can properly be addressed, if there's a reasonable expectation of their arising.

So, we have now gone through these considerations and have made the assessment as to what type of operating suite will be needed. Which surgical center(s) or hospital(s) we are able to choose from will now be dictated by the patient's insurance plan. This alone can be the determining factor regarding when and how to proceed. For if we are locked into a specific location, now we must find out what the *availability* is of the particular type of operating room/facility we need. Should the availability not be in sync with the patient's or surgeon's schedule, well, then, we get to start the whole time-consuming process over again. But let's add one more layer of complexity:

Urologic surgery can be done in one of three ways. First, we have our "open cases," meaning the procedure is performed through an open incision. This requires an operating room designed for such intervention. Next, there are laparoscopic and robotic assisted laparoscopic procedures. Laparoscopy is a type of minimally invasive surgery in which the procedure is performed through small incisions with extended instruments. For a robotic procedure, a robotic assisting device is utilized to improve dexterity/visualization for laparoscopic surgery. This mandates availability of the robot. Most hospitals have only one, possibly two (some large university settings might have three or more), since these instruments can cost up to two million dollars each. The instruments are shared by all surgeons, and having to factor in *their* schedules as well as the hospital's makes the process quite complex. Finally, the bulk of urologic surgery is performed endoscopically, meaning with instruments that are placed through the urethra, into the bladder, and if necessary up into the kidney or kidneys. The issue with this last type of procedure is that it requires a specific cystoscopy table, which is an operating table designed specifically for endoscopic procedures. It allows use of imaging at the same time as one is operating. Scheduling the right facility means having access not just to an operating room but to a specific room with specific equipment for a specific procedure—a room and equipment shared by numerous surgeons.

CHAPTER 4 | *The Illness of Medicine*

Assuming we have all agreed on a date and location and have received confirmation from the hospital or surgical center, the patient must now go through a list of instructions. There are limitations to what the patient can eat or drink and up to what time prior to surgery. Anesthesia induction (putting a patient to sleep) has the potential to cause regurgitation (vomiting), and given the circumstances, this can potentially lead to a severe complication involving the lungs, which is why strict adherence to the NPO (Latin abbreviation for *nothing per oral*) is required. The patients are informed of which drugs they are allowed to continue taking and which are to be discontinued prior to surgery, and when. Given NPO restrictions on the day of a procedure, diabetics, for instance, need to adjust their medications to prevent hypoglycemia (low blood sugar), which can be potentially quite dangerous. Medications taken for coronary artery disease or vascular conditions, such as aspirin and a variety of blood thinners, need to be stopped or their dosages modified. Any bowel preparation that needs to be accomplished prior to surgery requires explanation and review. Patients must also see their primary physician, and some will be required to have a cardiac evaluation/clearance. If the patient has other significant underlying medical conditions, this may mandate additional assessment. Obviously, all of this requires coordination and diligence to ensure that all of the parts of the equation are completed. Finally, and potentially the most aggravating issue of all, *authorization* from the all-important insurance company must often be obtained.

It is said that he who owns the gold makes the golden rules. In the case of medical care in the United States, it is the insurance companies that own the gold. Looking at the skyline, they seem to have the highest and largest buildings. Obtaining insurance-company approval for a surgical procedure can be difficult, for the insurers will not only "assess" the need for the procedure but will also determine the "appropriate" number of days the patient will be allowed to stay in the hospital, have rehabilitation services, etc. I'm not using scare quotes casually here. The fact is, the assessor deciding the appropriateness of the procedure is highly unlikely to be someone capable of *doing* the procedure, meaning the insurance approval "expert" is generally not a practicing physician in the area in which we are trying to get approval. Without understanding any of the nuances, the approval expert determines patient needs from a script of indications and possible interventions "allowed." Often, I have found that the medical directors of insurance companies are semi-retired or part-time physicians, perhaps of limited clinical experience. Certainly, most do not have equal training and expertise in each and every medical scenario on which they are rendering judgment. Yet they are the ones determining if a patient can undergo a particular treatment or procedure.

I clearly remember, as a surgical resident, seeing a middle-aged man walking gingerly down the hospital floor, pushing his IV (intravenous bag of fluid) pole alongside. He was wearing his hospital gown in the usual way, partially untied, allowing a full view of his overgrown posterior. He was moaning with each step. I recalled seeing him the previous days walking in the same hunched-over manner. I asked one of my fellow residents about this patient's history. He had undergone an uneventful (meaning uncomplicated) spinal laminectomy—surgery typically performed

CHAPTER 4 | *The Illness of Medicine*

to help alleviate pain from a spinal disc/vertebrae problem. Back then, patients were "allowed" to stay in the hospital three, possibly four days after this procedure. However, given his "particularly severe postoperative pain," he was staying longer—for an entire week. Everyone coming out of that procedure had the same pain. So why was he able to stay the week and get his requested intravenous morphine? He happened to be his HMO's medical director. Every other premium-paying patient in his HMO got denied additional days for pain, but since he was the director, well, no problem. Yes. Problem.

How and when did this all become so complicated? If reading this chapter about the process of obtaining treatment is making your head spin, imagine what it's like being the patient living through it. We need to examine this process more closely—look at the cracks and see where improvement can be made.

CHAPTER 5

Injectable Erections

Part of being a urologist means treating sexual dysfunction, and I noted through my years of practice that many men—regardless of age and relative health—would climb uphill, backwards, in high-heeled shoes, if it meant they could obtain or maintain a better erection.

Significant erectile-dysfunction research dates back well prior to the development of the ever-so-popular oral agents (Viagra, Cialis, Levitra, Stendra) that hit the market in the late 1990s and early 2000s. The physiology of vasodilation (the filling of blood vessels with blood) in the penis was being tested and subsequently manipulated by various drugs that could cause nearly immediate tumescence (engorgement of the penis). These drugs had previously been used for a variety of medical indications, but up until this point they had not been injected directly into the penis for the purpose of inducing an erection. A new era of treatment for sexual dysfunction was emerging. First used solely in experimental settings and as diagnostic tools for assessing the etiology of erectile dysfunction (at the time referred to as "impotence"), these vasoactive agents

CHAPTER 5 | The Illness of Medicine

(phentolamine, papaverine, prostaglandins) were eventually formulated for general patient prescription use. Patients were instructed by the urologists or staff on the proper means of injecting one's own penis with these drugs to achieve an erection on-demand. Initially, the patients needed to draw up the syringe, much as a diabetic would measure out and draw up his own syringe of insulin. With increased acceptance and use of this modality, combinations of the drugs became common as more information regarding dosage and safety became evident. Eventually, these drugs became commercially available in prepared combinations or preloaded syringes. The patient no longer had to measure, mix, or draw up his own drugs. Even various (previously unheard of) pharmacies began popping up and advertising their proprietary combinations for sale. ("Prescription only" was the mandate, but I still have my doubts as to how well this was regulated.)

Demand was high, and research and development continued on additional means of making these vasoactive drugs available to the penis. Another form of prostaglandins was being marketed under the brand name MUSE. This was an intra-urethral suppository, meaning that a man would insert it into the urethral opening of his penis. Eventual absorption would be followed by vasodilation and erection. The idea was to avoid having to insert a needle into one's penis to obtain an erection. The drug was expensive and some patients noted a penile and pelvic "ache" from the medication. Consequently, injectable agents continued to be popular.

Given patient demand, which drove potentially significant revenue, it was no surprise that a number of non-urologically trained physicians began prescribing these medications, some with rather limited experience of their side effects. A general rule in surgery is that if you can't manage the complication, then you shouldn't be performing the procedure. Similarly, from my point of care, if a physician doesn't understand or know how to manage the complications of a drug, then he or she should not prescribe it.

As the lax prescribing of these drugs increased, so too did the frequency with which emergency rooms would contact the urologist on call for help when a patient would present with problems related to the penile application of vasoactive drugs—bruising or bleeding from a poorly placed needle, pain at an injection site, or possibly a skin infection from poor injection technique. However, the most dreaded of these ER calls involved a condition known as priapism—that is, a prolonged erection that won't go down. These calls tended to come at the most inopportune times—in the middle of the night or on weekends. In my experience, the patients who came in for priapism after a vasoactive drug injection were generally of two types: those whose physicians had limited understanding of its effects and an inability to manage complications, and those who obtained the drug for recreational use. By "recreational use," I mean patients for whom the drug was never prescribed. These individuals often had no erectile problems but simply wanted to use the drug for sexual amplification. These individuals would at times be sharing syringes and having orgies with multiple partners over an extended period of time. Others would state they were "experimenting". Patients would inject themselves or—as was often the case—the drug would be obtained and injected by a

CHAPTER 5 | *The Illness of Medicine*

"friend," meaning someone the patient had just met at the party. After hours of an erection—often many, uncomfortable hours, leading to severe pain—the patient would come in for help. The stories were always more or less the same: "I didn't really know the guy injecting me." "He told me it was safe." And so on. At the hospitals where I practiced, many of the recreational users were HIV+ and often stoned, drunk, or on a variety of additional illicit drugs at the time they were injected.

The most significant problem with priapism is, potentially, it causing such damage to the penis that genuine and profound erectile dysfunction can ensue. Treatment of priapism carries similar risk. For the patient being treated, the likelihood of *permanent* erectile dysfunction is now very real. This was always delineated clearly before treatment was even initiated. Often this was when the patients realized their absolute stupidity in allowing this event to occur. This would be the moment they sobered up. You could see it in their faces. They started paying attention to what was being said to them: "Damage to the penis may be permanent either from the extended erection or from the treatment." No longer were the less distressed patients proudly showing off their protuberant penis. If they'd assumed they were in for a simple fix—a misconception probably encouraged by their injecting friend—they were now fully aware of their folly.

For the urologist being called in, this was an insult to his practice and life. The time and effort needed to detumesce, or reduce the erection, could be quite significant. The procedure was also unavoidably bloody. This put everyone in the treatment bay at risk for any communicable diseases the often intoxicated, needle-sharing patient had brought into their lives. Hepatitis was common as well as HIV, a shared needle often being a great transmitter of disease. So the urologist, being on the front line of this activity, puts himself at serious risk for contamination or infection. And the following morning, after being up all night taking care of the condition, the doctor must tend to his office hours or scheduled surgeries.

In order to reduce the erection, we would generally start by injecting medications into the penis that would reverse the effect of the vasodilators previously injected by the patient or his erstwhile friend. This would be done in combination with techniques of aspiration and irrigation (inserting a large-bore needle into the penis, physically drawing out the clotted blood, and then irrigating the corporal bodies, which are the paired areas of the penis that become engorged with blood during an erection). Often this was quite painful, and on occasion needed to be supplemented by various surgical procedures to drain the penis—the supplemental procedures sometimes mandating a trip to the operating room. It was a long, difficult night for all involved. Many times the outcome was less than desired, and the procedure was a bloody mess to clean up after whether or not it was a success.

In my experience, when we were successful, we typically never saw the patient again and just as typically never received payment for services. If the treatment was unsuccessful and the patient never regained erectile activity, it was always a problem. Those patients would come back to be seen, and were often quite remorseful,

CHAPTER 5 | *The Illness of Medicine*

exhibiting none of the swagger that some of the more intoxicated patients had initially demonstrated in the ER. All were anxious, and for good reason. Most often, the only treatment left to try was the implanting of a penile prosthesis. This is a silicone mechanical device, usually inflatable, placed in the part of the penis where engorgement would normally occur. The device generally works quite well. But needing a prosthetic erection is not a desirable outcome from a moment of being irresponsible with your body.

Medications for erectile activity were a genuine pharmaceutical advancement abused by those merely looking for an all-nighter. It was really an insult to be involved in treating the majority of these self-inflicted complications. If you need the injectable medications, they do work. And when prescribed and monitored properly by a knowledgeable physician, they can be a safe and effective form of treatment. But as with the party-goer submitting to injection from a dubious friend, even legitimate patients should be wary of the immediate fix that some clinics advertise. There is no rapid cure for a complex problem such as erectile dysfunction. To find the proper treatment and solution can take multiple sessions involving various drugs, dosages, and proper instruction. Don't be in a hurry to get that damn erection—the consequences of a mistake in treatment, or self-management of the condition, can be devastating.

CHAPTER 6

Technology

I know it sounds cliché when the older generation reflects on the current state of affairs and feels that the olden days were better. I think in the case of medicine, it is true. Yes, there have been significant improvements through our technology. We have better instrumentation, improved diagnostic capabilities, a more refined understanding of physiology, and greater ability to intervene with disease processes.

But I feel the situation is somewhat analogous to the current state of interpersonal communication. Today we have fax machines, text messaging, email, voicemail. Do we communicate any better? I would argue not. In fact, I think because of these options, we have found ways to communicate without really talking to one another. As a consequence of our technological improvements in communication, we have reduced that communication to brief decontextualized bursts of information—information that is subject to potential misinterpretation and misunderstanding. Instead of picking up the phone to discuss an issue, we "discuss" via typing, and how many text messages have been interpreted by the recipient in a way never intended by the sender?

CHAPTER 6 | The Illness of Medicine

The same has occurred in medicine. Given the ease of access provided by a computer (or smartphone), why bother to call the referring M.D. to discuss a patient or problem? Why should I stay on hold as the doctor's staff tries to locate him or pull him out of an exam room? It's easier simply to send an email. By the time it's read, however, the patient may have left the office, or the situation may have evolved a bit beyond the original concern. A game of email tag now begins. And what would have been a simple call and discussion now becomes a drawn-out process. Oh, for the good ole days of just picking up the telephone.

Our technology has also forged new roads of confusion and concern among our patients. There once was a time when a patient in need could call the office after-hours for concerns about a new or ongoing problem. The answering service would call or page the M.D. Patients often do not have that as an option today: the answering services are computerized. A patient calling the physician's office is then connected to a messaging center that undoubtedly gives a multiple-choice list of prompts to which the caller must respond. Urology is a field that is often dealing with the elderly, many of whom simply cannot adapt to the communication changes or do not understand the mechanism for reaching their physician. Consequently, their calls are lost or improperly routed through the labyrinthine answering system, or the patients simply hang up in confusion. Their problem, unaddressed, is left to progress in the interim.

Among other technological wonders in the world of medicine are the now mandated "portal systems," by which patients can access their medical records online 24/7. The patients can be sitting at home and decide to read their recent lab results—not necessarily understanding them, but they have this option. This usually leads to their next move, which is to write the doctor on the portal system, questioning the results. Few patients wait until their upcoming appointment to go over labs, because technology today has enabled—even encouraged—our desire for instant knowledge and feedback.

I can understand why the patients call. Having just tried to interpret data without understanding any of the intricacies simply leads to anxiety, confusion, and frustration on their part. The patients read something they don't understand, or certain lab values are highlighted (often inconsequentially), and they become alarmed. This prompts a call, typically in the evening, when most patients return home from work. Others elect to page the doctor (pronto) to discuss the issue. This happens day or night, weekday or weekend. For the physician, it becomes a never-ending list of calls to return, typically for only slight, harmless deviations from "normal" on lab results—deviations that have his patients concerned. This fatigues the doctor, both mentally and physically, leading to his or her frustration and ultimately to fewer calls being returned on his or her part. The anxiety of the patient grows. The cycle of frustration continues on both ends—for patient and for doctor. Frustration leads to anger.

However, I think the most significant change in patient access to health care information has involved the internet in general, which is filled with innumerable sites related to health care,

CHAPTER 6 | *The Illness of Medicine*

each with countless links to still more such sites—the lot of them offering bounteous medical verbiage for the interpretation or misinterpretation of all who click in. I suspect the vast majority of sites are well intended and overseen by true expert advisors. Unfortunately, in addition to possessing often limited powers of interpretation, many patients can't separate the reliable sites from the more fringe ones.

I once had a patient present through the emergency room with an abscessed scrotum and significant scrotal cellulitis. This is an infection of the scrotum that if not tended to promptly and appropriately can lead to a serious, life-threatening condition known as necrotizing fasciitis. The patient was febrile (meaning he had a fever), and his scrotum was strawberry-red and enlarged to the size of a cantaloupe. Incidentally, the patient was HIV+. He was also in miserable pain from the swelling and infection. When questioned, he explained in detail how/when/where this all started: with the internet.

Apparently, the patient had decided he wanted a larger scrotum, and had found a how-to online. I witnessed quite a few unusual things practicing urology in the Viagra and internet era. The most bizarre and self-mutilating activities I came across in hospital emergency rooms often, if not always, involved the male genitals. I'm sure psychiatrists have an understanding of this behavior and an explanation for its relative frequency. But reading about it in a scholarly journal or discussing it at a conference with coffee in hand is significantly different from being on the front lines taking care of it. I do believe that in any analysis of why such bizarre behavior occurs, consideration must be given both to people's internet access and to their inability (or reluctance) to separate normal medical recommendations from those that are more outré. People apparently believe what they read online, often for no more reason than that they want to believe it.

This patient who'd desired a more endowed scrotum had read an online article that described, in detail, how to go about achieving such a thing. Despite the current agony in his nether regions, he even went excitedly to his knapsack and pulled out the instructions he'd downloaded and printed from the internet. He was visibly stunned that I'd never heard of such a "therapy" and that I wasn't interested in reading his "article." My lack of knowledge and curiosity seemed to shatter his confidence in me as a medical professional. After all, that he'd found this technique on the internet was, to him, proof of its very legitimacy, and he assured me that he had followed the instructions to the letter: He used a large-bore needle with a large syringe to inject two tubes' worth of lubricating jelly. Each tube, obtained at the local grocery store, was 120cc in volume—a total of 240cc. For comparison's sake, a can of Coke is 355cc. He injected the jelly into his scrotum to enhance the volume within his pants. Certainly, his technique was far from sterile and his final volume of enhancement was arrived at merely by his running out of lubricant. His sources for the needles and syringe were almost certainly questionable as well. I once had a patient present to the ER with a similar type of infection of his penis, after he had "read" somewhere online about crushing Viagra tablets, mixing the powder with water, and then injecting the "sludge." I'm sure the reader can imagine where this led. Nothing good came of it.

CHAPTER 6 | The Illness of Medicine

Now, there is much more good than bad online. There are highly reputable sites giving excellent information that can be trusted and used for patient education. These sites promote a more informed decision by the patient regarding a condition or treatment. But again, knowing which information is applicable, how much is too much, and when to turn off the monitor is difficult to ascertain. I had many patients over the years who relied so much on websites and chat rooms that they were confrontational when in the office to discuss their problem. They presumed a certain expertise because they'd spent several hours or days glued to medical websites. They now knew a bit of the vocabulary, but without understanding the true meaning of the words they were so proudly quoting in the office. I may have treated prostate cancer for nearly thirty years, day in and day out. But after a few hours online, some of my patients were now dictating to me diagnoses and treatment plans based on what some internet so-and-so had said or recommended.

I support self-education and encourage patients to learn about their conditions. But a little bit of knowledge, without a complete grasp of the context and processes involved, can lead to misunderstandings that are potentially dangerous.

I had a patient with prostate cancer approximately fifteen years ago who was a very wealthy individual from an affluent suburb. He even went so far as to tell me once that he felt "his" physicians served him, and therefore we were like employees to him. I dreaded our office appointments. He was never verbally abusive, but he always behaved as if he were the one in control. I was there to take his orders. He disagreed with my recommendation for treatment, which was a radical prostatectomy (surgical removal of the prostate gland). This patient claimed he had "done his homework," and was convinced that an alternative treatment he'd read about on the internet was best for him. I pleaded with him not to go into the realm of herbal treatment that he "knew" would work. But he left my practice and sought out doctors across the country (money was no object) who would proceed with this type of therapy. Again, not all cancers of the same organ behave identically. Patients often will compare treatments with their friends, or with things they've read online, while not truly grasping the subtle but consequential differences.

This patient returned to me three years later. His cancer had now metastasized (spread outside the confines of the prostate) into his bones and lymph nodes. For the first time, he looked at me with eyes that revealed sadness, defeat. He knew his decision had been wrong. This time he listened to me. He didn't interrupt me as I spoke, as he had done previously. He didn't quote articles or scholars of the sort he had so vehemently defended in the past. He just listened.

And after our discussion, he simply looked up at me and said, "Doc, I just should have listened to you."

Not that I know all, because I clearly don't. But I dealt with a defined group of medical problems on a daily basis for years. I could see the disease progression coming, and I knew where it was going. I simply asked that the patient respect that experience. Respect your doctor's knowledge. If you don't, then find another doctor. And keep the internet in its place. It's only a reference site. It's not a provider.

CHAPTER 7

The Seventh Floor

I knew I'd been in practice a long time when I could walk down the rehabilitation floor in one of the hospitals and realize I knew quite a few of the older patients on the floor. I remembered when they were younger, which meant I was getting older too. But some had had a head start, or perhaps they just hadn't had very good luck in life, and their diseases accelerated the aging process.

But going onto the rehabilitation floor at this particular hospital also made me aware of many of the problems at the hospital that I was becoming increasingly frustrated with. Many of the patients on this floor were now past the acute phases of their illnesses. Cardiac patients, for instance, were now engaged in increased activity. Patients with neurological ailments were undergoing occupational, speech, or physical therapy. All of the patients were gradually resuming independence, but at different stages, and for different medical conditions. As a consequence of these significant differences, life on the floor seemed disjointed. Each patient was up and about doing his or her own thing. This also made evident to me the significant changes occurring in nursing care.

CHAPTER 7 | *The Illness of Medicine*

I was quietly making my rounds one Thursday afternoon on the seventh floor, alongside the hospital urology nurse practitioner. NPs, as they are sometimes referred to, are an invaluable asset to managing one's practice. These are nurses with advanced training, and they can truly facilitate patient care. I have rarely met NPs that weren't competent and dedicated. They can perform many of our fundamental floor procedures, and they often communicate effectively with patients regarding health conditions and treatment plans—thus bridging the abyss between physicians and patients. Perhaps most important, they are able to interact very efficiently with the floor nurses. A good NP is a highly valuable asset.

Unfortunately, my experience with the majority of floor nurses was one of slow but steady decline. I don't believe it had to do with a lack of dedication or interest in health care on their part. Many nurses I encountered truly wanted to make a difference and improve the delivery of health care to patients. But the hospital "system" had gotten in the way. Floor nurses are now spending more time at computer terminals documenting what has transpired in their patient encounters than actually developing an understanding of patients' diseases and processes. Simply put, less time is being spent with the actual patient.

There was a time early in my practice when I could call a floor nurse to evaluate a patient's condition. I would ask not only for the most recent vital signs (blood pressure, heart rate, respiratory rate, and temperature), but could also inquire if the patient was sick. How did the patient look? Did he appear in distress or in pain? Was he calm or anxious? How did the abdomen feel—was it soft or distended? The floor nurses twenty years ago could answer these questions without missing a beat. I could readily rely on their interpretation of a patient's condition. It helped dictate when I would come into the hospital to make rounds and might compel me to change my daily routine for a potential problem that was evolving in a particular patient.

Today's hospital nurse is quite good at relaying basic data. He or she could obviously convey vital signs to the surgeon over the phone. After all, the temperature is measured by an instrument. Blood pressure is measured by another instrument. But if the nurse were to be asked how the patient looked, there would be a pause, a hesitation, as if the question didn't compute with their preprogrammed available responses, as if it were out of their range to be able to effectively say whether or not the patient looked ill.

"Is the abdomen soft or distended?" I would ask.

"I don't know what you mean," the nurse would respond.

"Okay, well, does the belly look full and tense like a drum?"

"I guess so" —said without conviction or confidence.

"Can you feel a pulse in the ankle," I once asked.

"What do you mean?" the nurse replied. "Where should I look for it?"

"Really ..." (I could think of no other response.)

And the conversation would continue in this fashion.

Is it the floor nurses' fault? Not really. The modern nurse has been taught primarily to observe and document, to notify a physician

CHAPTER 7 | The Illness of Medicine

should something appear significantly out of line. But detecting subtleties and identifying when conditions are in a state of flux, before they become so obvious that even a novice could pick up a change in the patient's status, are no longer skills the modern floor nurse has had to cultivate.

The floor nurse is overworked, poorly supported, and not trained anymore to interpret. Unfortunately, in many instances, his or her job has been reduced to relaying data.

Personally, I don't care that the nurse has spent hours documenting that the call-light button is within reach of the patient and that the guardrails are up. Yes, yes, these are important in our ever more litigious health care environment. But could someone please just tell me how the patient "looks"? Unlikely.

* * * * * * * * * *

So, the nurse practitioner and I were making our rounds on the seventh floor—where rehabilitation was in full force—when I saw one of my partner's patients in the hallway, a ninety-year-old admitted for a urinary-tract and scrotal infection. He had been in the hospital for over a week and was now feeling quite well. He spent his days riding around the hospital floor in a red electric cart, colliding with staff and fellow patients alike (including me) while on a quest to find one of his hospitalized buddies.

We walked into the room of my patient, an eighty-six-year-old recovering from what was initially an outpatient inguinal hernia procedure. This operation is performed to correct a defect or a weakness in the fascia, a supporting tissue of our body. In this particular case, the structural support was deficient in the inguinal area allowing the abdominal contents to "bulge" adjacent to his scrotum. One of the significant changes in medicine in recent years has been the conversion of the majority of surgical procedures from inpatient to outpatient operations. Translation: patients now tend to go home on the same day as their surgery. The days of typically being in the hospital for weeks (or long ago, even months) following surgery are long gone. Unfortunately, this puts considerable strain on the patients and their families, as healing still takes time. The difficulty of simply getting out of bed to go to the washroom can be considerable. Multiply this problem for eating and bathing. Also, having to change surgical dressings after early hospital discharge is both frightening and difficult for most spouses or other family caregivers. This particular patient had had his hernia repaired. But during the surgery a problem occurred, and he subsequently was required to have part of his colon removed. So much for the outpatient-surgery plan. I was seeing him because along the way, his bladder gave out as well, and now he was in urinary retention—that is, he couldn't pee.

As we walked out of the room, I was again nearly run over by our ninety-year-old NASCAR racer, driving his little red electric cart. I think the nurses had given up scolding him. He was out of control.

I then encountered another old patient. He was in for rehabilitation after a hip replacement. The physical therapist was walking behind him closely as he took gingerly steps with the aid of a walker. My mind flashed back to when he was a patient of mine, nearly twenty years before.

CHAPTER 7 | *The Illness of Medicine*

I remembered it so clearly. The man was sixty when we first met. A blood test had revealed that he had an elevated prostate-specific antigen (PSA), a possible indicator of cancer of the prostate gland. (Although the PSA test has had its critics, it is a very useful benchmarking tool for urologists, helping both to identify patients with prostate cancer and to observe possible progression of the cancer over time). I performed a biopsy of his prostate and determined, unfortunately, that he indeed had prostate cancer. Although the cancer was treatable, the patient's wife, in her hysterics, was not. She was by far the most difficult patient spouse I ever had to deal with. I spent hours and hours on the telephone trying to console, educate, and instruct her regarding her husband's condition. Seeing them as a couple in the office often meant I had to cancel everything afterward, including my dinner that night and possibly breakfast the following morning. She was not only impossible to control but also unkind and antagonistic.

Finally, after what seemed like an eternity of discussing options, they elected for a type of radiation therapy whereby small radioactive "seeds" are placed into the prostate gland as a means of managing the cancer. This treatment, otherwise known as brachytherapy, is highly effective and generally tolerated quite well. It involves the urologist, often in combination with a radiation oncologist, inserting into the perineum (the region between the scrotum and anus) small needles through which radioactive seeds (or pellets) are inserted into the prostate gland. The seeds are about the size of a piece of rice, and they emanate radioactivity for variable lengths of time to destroy the cancer. Most men will have active radiation for months after the seeds are placed. The actual seeds are left in the prostate and are never removed. After they have done their job, the metallic shell of the now exhausted radioactive implant will remain in place for the duration of the patient's life.

This was the treatment the patient decided to undergo—after literally months of deliberation and discussion regarding the risks and benefits of the various treatment options. Finally, when the procedure was performed, all went flawlessly. No apparent complications occurred, and we hoped for a cure. I was elated simply to be done. With any luck, the two-hour phone conversations would dwindle as the patient recuperated, and normal life in my office would again resume.

Then, four weeks later, a complication occurred—one I could not have predicted in two lifetimes, one I'd never had happen before (or after, for that matter). But of course it had to happen to her, and it did—literally.

My patient and his wife were having sex, which was allowed, but only with a condom at this stage of the recuperation. That part of the postoperative sex instruction (wearing a condom), however, was not followed. Given the specific act they were engaged in, it might not have seemed necessary. At any rate, a radioactive seed must have dislodged, and during oral sex, she swallowed it.

Her husband, my patient, was fine—and happy as a lark. He was cured, and he was getting oral sex. She was beyond a mess.

Long story short, I think I aged a few years in the weeks that followed, but she did fine and he did fine. And I continued my little walk down the hallway with the nurse, reminiscing about the good old days.

CHAPTER 8

The Hospital Room

I remember my first overnight-camp experience. I must have been about ten years old. I was in a cabin that smelled of old rotten wood. The mattress I was assigned had probably been made during the Civil War, and the light source was a single incandescent bulb that jiggled each time the cabin door was opened or closed—giving the room a strange, eerie effect at night. The windows were stuck, and in the Indiana summer heat, the room temperature never seemed to get below the mid-eighties. It was hot. The other campers were just a mean bunch of kids, and I really hated jumping into that damn freezing pool each day to play a game that made no sense. It was not a good time. I wanted to go home, to be with my dog and to run around in familiar surroundings with my friends. It was sort of like being a patient in the hospital.

Hospitals are strange places. Patients are usually there involuntarily, unless they came in to have, for instance, major elective cosmetic surgery. And even then, they want to get out as soon as possible. The rooms are generally small, with nothing but a thin, non-sound-resistant curtain separating you from the stranger lying in the same

CHAPTER 8 | *The Illness of Medicine*

room five feet away. I think the curtains are made by the same folks who designed the hospital gown, both being almost completely useless. The curtain can never be pulled around you for complete visual separation. Somehow the eyelets at the top of the curtain seem to catch on the hooks, so the curtain will draw only halfway. Despite there being two patients in most hospital rooms, there is only one sink and one box of disposable gloves. "Oh, good morning, sir," the nurse might say as part of the morning ritual. "Don't mind me while I just grab some gloves and now go see your neighbor."

The little tray tables patients are supposed to stow their belongings in/eat on/keep the phone on/keep their books on/etc. are way overburdened. Also, they don't really roll. I think the wheels are sold to the hospital already broken. Furthermore, lifting the tray table from a low to a high position will typically wrench your back, and how is the patient expected to do it him-or herself while lying in bed? What kind of genius invented this, and how come it keeps being manufactured in the same malfunctioning way? I did not see one design improvement on the hospital tray table in nearly thirty years.

The lighting design of the typical hospital bed is also ingenious. First, the switch by the door is never labeled. Consequently, when making early morning rounds, the nurse (or doctor) will inevitably (if innocently) illuminate the light above the wrong patient. This will further add to the joy each patient feels when his or her little space is violated—again.

The hospital bed is an interesting invention. It requires about a week's stay to fully understand each bed's little quirks. "Oh, if you want to turn on the light," the nurse says, "you need to push the button twice—

no, not that one. The other one. No, that one controls the reading light. You want to push this button to turn on the main exam light." And so it goes every morning on rounds. Getting the bed to go up and down usually works well enough. It's figuring out how to raise the head and not the feet that requires an advanced degree. And what is with those pillows? Hospital pillows are anything but soft. They are obviously industrial in design and could double as sandbags during a flood.

I have never seen the patient whose bed is next to the window have window coverings that fully open or close. But by the third day in the hospital, most patients are so desensitized to privacy—what with the hospital gown that just flies open with minimal movement, and the patient's having undergone multiple rectal exams and an enema or suppository or two for the inevitable constipation—that they couldn't care less about the neighbors looking in. All privacy is forfeited. All concern regarding privacy subsequently falls away as well. The patient who came into the hospital prim and proper leaves with a renewed understanding of decency.

No conversation can be held in private. It doesn't matter if your doctor is telling you about a cantaloupe-sized tumor that is now growing in your abdomen. It doesn't matter if he is telling you about the risks of tomorrow's brain surgery, including your probable loss of reasoning and judgment. Any phone conversation is heard by four ears, not only your two. Just move on, undergo your treatment, and whoever hears your conversations in the meantime, well, let them.

And if one needs a bedside procedure? Oh, my. Listening to your roommate undergo the placement of a nasogastric tube (a tube inserted through the nose and into the stomach) or the placement of

CHAPTER 8 | *The Illness of Medicine*

a Foley catheter (a tube inserted into the bladder) is most unpleasant, particularly when the placement isn't going well. No pillow can block out the noise enough. And this is to say nothing of the perhaps audible discomfort the patient must have been experiencing that prompted the need for these interventions in the first place.

One unique thing about being in the hospital is all the visitors you have. The nurses come in every several hours to pass medications, to make sure your catheter (the tube in your bladder) is not being suspended around your neck, and to confirm that your needs are being met. But don't bother using the little button next to your bed to call them. They are overworked, with too many patients to look after. Nurses today have a phonebook's worth of documentation to do—most of it being without genuine medical purpose or need. But again, in order for the hospital to be paid, and for legal issues to be avoided, documentation must be performed. Whoever assigned the actual tasks that require such detailed record keeping must never have actually *been in the hospital,* or he or she would realize that such documentary nonsense is actually preventing nurses from tending to patients' incessant calls for... the nurse!

You will get to meet the dietary personnel, however. They're going to visit you six times a day. You will have your meal tray delivered, and then you will have it removed—three hours later. (Oh yes, and with the tray table in front of you littered with your inedible meal, you are stuck in that bed.) It doesn't matter that you ordered pasta and received steak instead. They actually taste the same.

More than likely a social worker will visit you, assigned to make sure you have proper follow-up after your discharge. These individuals work quite hard, and will stop in probably several times a day with updates. Mostly they will come bearing bad news for you to mull over between visits (e.g., the outpatient care facility won't accept your insurance, or the one you need is in the next county). But not to worry, they will keep you updated.

If you require physical therapy, occupational therapy, respiratory therapy, or—best of all—a combination of the above, well, more visitation. But your day is not through yet. Yes, you are supposed to get your rest (after all, you are healing), but the pesky housekeeper needs to mop your room, clean the sink, and tidy up. Also, your physician or his or her designee will be checking up, possibly multiple times. And if you are in a teaching institution, you might have the opportunity to repeat your medical history at least three times a day—once to the physician or designee, once to a medical student or students, and once possibly even to a nursing student. Or do you repeat it three times a day specifically to the medical student? I guess you just stop counting. The phlebotomist may come in—again—this time with her boss, because that vein in your hand that she tapped at 5:00 a.m., well, sorry, it didn't provide enough of a sample. And the bloodletting needs to be repeated. Next time, just hope they don't send in the rookie.

And did you ever think about where all those visitors have been *before* they came into your room? Maybe in the room down the hall where that inevitable poor patient could be heard hacking all night? Maybe they just came from the room with the patient recovering from hepatitis, pancreatitis, conjunctivitis, appendicitis, colitis… Who knows what "-itis" they were near, and is now in your space.

CHAPTER 8 | *The Illness of Medicine*

And finally, let's not forget your family, who will come in to keep you company (as if you need it). My experience was that most families came in groups—often exceeding the maximum number of allowable visitors. No mind, nobody is really counting anyway. Unfortunately, the number of chairs in your half of the room is exactly half of what is needed. Your kin start colonizing the window ledge. And guess what? They brought you dinner! Now it's a party—just the thing to top off an exhausting day of poking, prodding, explaining, and re-explaining. After a full day of tests, exams, and having IVs replaced, all you really want is to be left alone, in the dark. After all, you are sick.

The family-sized bucket of fried chicken is now at your feet. Napkins are flying and tempers are flaring, as nobody has any room to sit and the anxiety surrounding your medical condition has just got everyone in a bit of a tizzy. Questions are being asked. It's really lovely to see everyone together—except it's in your hospital room. You have a catheter draining your urine for all to observe (even little Johnny, who won't stop commenting on your bodily functions and who keeps a close eye on your urine output). You are tired, and all you really want is to be alone. Finally, at the witching hour of 8:00 p.m., the usual family deportation time, you are relieved of company. Except for one person: the roommate.

During my time practicing medicine, I concluded that the hospital-roommate situation was inversely related to the compatibility of the occupants. If one was quiet, the other snored like a beast. If one was in for a bowel obstruction, the other would be having diarrhea. One liked the TV on all night, while the other desired silence. I don't think the hospital could have achieved better incompatibility with a plan for exactly that outcome.

If it weren't for the patients being ill, I would say that such issues would probably be tolerated much better. But patients in the hospital are not at their best. They are tired, scared, even traumatized by the events and procedures they are undergoing. They are disturbed all day, and awakened all night for vital-sign checks. The patients actually cannot get the rest required simply to get well. The roommate who coughs all night, the roommate who is up screaming in pain all night, does not facilitate the process of healing. And this describes the situation in a private hospital. I can recall during my residency treating patients at the Veterans Administration (VA) hospital. In some VA facilities, many patients are not in rooms but in wards, with four to six patients in a ward together. The problems outlined previously are simply multiplied.

So it is no wonder patients are eager to be discharged as quickly as possible. The hospital room is not a sanctum of healing. It is a room packed with too much activity, too much commotion, and too little opportunity for the patient to actually rest. Newer, more lucrative institutions are now building more private rooms—but again, all that does is eliminate the roommate variable. This will not prevent the phlebotomist from missing the vein, or forestall the constant nursing interactions, many of which are purely for documenting purposes rather than for actual medical need. The rolling barrage of students, therapists, and aids coming in ostensibly to help makes the hospital room a difficult place to be. Better to get out ASAP!

CHAPTER 9

Viagra, and Things

I must admit, the development of the class of drugs known as phosphodiesterase 5 inhibitors, or PDE5i, is remarkable. This is the group of drugs used to enhance or prolong an erection. The brand names of such medications include Viagra, Cialis, Levitra, and Stendra. They have truly revolutionized the manner in which we both understand and treat erectile dysfunction.

The medication essentially works by inhibiting the breakdown of a substance produced in the lining of penile blood vessels, which causes vasodilation, which thereby increases the inflow of blood into the corpus cavernosum (spongy tissue) in the penis. Outflow is reduced by venous compression, and basically, with more inflow than outflow, engorgement of the penis proceeds and an erection occurs. The discovery of PDE5i completely changed the quality of life for the aging, sexually active male.

Viagra was the first of this class to be FDA approved and released, in the spring of 1998. I remember this time clearly; the phones in my office were ringing off the hook. Primary care physicians were uncomfortable prescribing these newly released drugs, yet people

CHAPTER 9 | *The Illness of Medicine*

were curious and many wanted the drug regardless of whether they actually needed it. Patients were scrambling for it while insurance companies were trying to figure out how to minimize their costs by placing limits on how many pills a patient could have in a given prescription. I have no doubt that some very serious statistical analyses were being performed, with devilishly clever statisticians hired by the insurance industry to calculate these limits and costs.

One of the more challenging questions that came up frequently during many initial male office evaluations, just as I was placing my hand on the door handle saying "goodbye," was the topic of erectile dysfunction. More than likely, it's what the patient really wanted to come in for in the first place. After first indicating that all was well in that area of life, somehow, many new patients would take the plunge, at the very end of the appointment, and reveal that things really weren't fine after all. Men will have the issue of an erection on their mind to their dying breath. I'm sure there are volumes of psychiatric textbooks dedicated to analyzing this topic. Perhaps it's due to the prevalence of television advertising for erectile-dysfunction treatment. Or possibly to the ads that are seen on every other page in most men's magazines. Add to those the effect of radio advertising for treatment centers that can give anyone an erection on their "first visit." We are simply inundated with the potential of having an erection, on demand, at whatever age. Patients with portable oxygen canisters, who come into the office and can barely walk let alone breathe after taking a few steps, all want to know about drugs or therapy to improve their erections. Since the 1998 introduction of Viagra, these discussions have become as regular as reviewing one's bowel habits. I think it has really gotten out of hand, and away from any apparent limit on practicality or need. Direct consumer advertising has done exactly what the pharmaceutical industry has asked of it: it has created the need.

Those television commercials promoting erectile-dysfunction treatment drive me nuts. In your average one-minute ad, two-thirds of the commercial is devoted to reviewing the risks of the drug. None of that information is heard and processed. Then again, when you tell someone that everything from flatulence to death can occur, most will just ignore the information. Men would come into the office literally demanding their "free sample" of whatever drug they saw last night at midnight on television, and they would shop around until someone gave them their sample, despite all rational discussion on why they shouldn't take it. Again, patients would go to the internet and dig up some article supporting their claim of need. The physician had been designated in these instances a mere dispenser of a preordained prescription, not a person with the medical expertise to decide which prescriptions were (or were not) appropriate. Why not just go to a vending machine?

* * * * * * * * * *

I once had a patient who was a CEO of a rather prominent company in the Chicago area. He was fifty-five and was experiencing what he described as "sexual dysfunction." Upon further discussion of this matter, he revealed that he had a wonderful, loving relationship with his wife. She was twenty years younger and a retired fashion model. He told me that given his extraordinary wealth, she could

CHAPTER 9 | *The Illness of Medicine*

have whatever money would buy. In turn, he could have sex as often as desired. Sounded like a true loving relationship to me. His concern was that given his age, he was no longer able to have sex three times a day—it was down to a measly two times a day. This, a tragedy of obviously epic proportions, is what preoccupied him, and in order to increase his performance, he was willing to take medication. I sincerely feel there is a societal problem present when this is why patients come to seek medical care.

Fortunately, I was well positioned at the time to get involved in this mad dash. During my residency, I'd begun performing standup comedy at local clubs. I took lessons on comedy delivery and found it both challenging and extremely rewarding. Little did I know the lessons learned would find their way into my urology practice a decade later. The pharmaceutical industry needed people to present information on PDE5i—both to the public and to potential prescribing physicians. I was paid by several pharmaceutical companies to give lectures and presentations to help disseminate the hows and whys of this new class of medication. Public speaking was never a problem for me, but with my newly gained experiences delivering standup, addressing both professional and nonprofessional groups was even easier. I was giving an informative lecture almost weekly. Once FDA approval was granted for Cialis and Levitra, well, it was game on! The competition among the companies was intense. I just kept giving those lectures to community groups, cardiologists, primary care physicians—just about anybody who would listen.

But the drugs started a medical dilemma that I hadn't seen before. Just by virtue of their availability, a need for them was created. Twenty-five-year-old patients would come into the office complaining of "erectile dysfunction" if they'd once lost an erection prematurely. Patients in their mid-eighties, who previously would have accepted the consequences of aging, were now demanding prescriptions for these new drugs. Much of the "need" was simply the consequence of brilliant marketing by the pharmaceutical industry. People watching television or reading magazines or newspapers were bombarded with advertisements regarding erectile dysfunction. A delicate subject that used to be discussed only in the doctor's office had now become part of candid, casual discussions around the company water cooler.

Understand, these were still real drugs. There were risks, possible complications, and potentially serious side effects. Overexertion for individuals not used to having sex could induce a myocardial infarction (heart attack). There'd already been reports of gastrointestinal issues, back pain, serious visual and auditory effects. The potential for priapism, which is a prolonged erection (one that lasts for hours), was not insignificant. This condition may lead to permanent erectile dysfunction. But these were all of little concern to patients on a quest for "The Erection".

Unfortunately, there was no filter regarding who would be exposed to information about the once sensitive subject of impotency and its treatment. Erectile function and dysfunction were everywhere, bombarding our airwaves, splashed across our printed media.

CHAPTER 9 | The Illness of Medicine

Another significant "side effect"—never considered amid the media blitz—was that children can also read, and watch. I'm quite sure young ones had questions, and didn't grasp what was or was not appropriate dinner conversation in many households. I can only imagine the questions they asked and the answers they were given.

Billboards with PDE5i content began popping up in the mid-2000s. Who didn't know "the little blue pill"? Everyone knew that seeing two people in adjacent ceramic white bathtubs was the Cialis promotion. Levitra ads featured a jock throwing a football through a tire swing.

The advertising on television was becoming quite annoying. Direct consumer advertising was not only increasing sales of the drugs but also, again, promoting the need for them. For the first time I could recall, men, rather than rejecting the possibility of their being afflicted with disease, were openly acknowledging they had one!

No man in the history of the world till then would ever have confessed to another that his erections were anything but stellar. The Penis was the appendage at the center of how many men defined themselves. The Greek god Priapus (with his enormous phallus) would be frowning down on our current male society if he were to see what was going on.

A medical definition of erectile dysfunction: "The inability to obtain or maintain an erection on a consistent basis for satisfactory completion of sexual activity." The social definition, however, had come to mean something much different. Now, anyone who couldn't obtain or maintain an erection for even one night was clamoring to get into the office to be seen and treated. Patients were pleading with our receptionist to get appointments ASAP. No matter how much an individual had had to drink, or how much a lack of sleep might have been affecting him, or how much stress he'd been under, any erection that had eluded him was proof of pathology, and he "deserved" to be treated. Age was no longer a limiting factor in the mind of the American male. He had been shown on TV that an erection was not a privilege, it was a right. And he wanted to exercise his.

I had young "patients" coming in because they hadn't been able to perform adequately on just one or two occasions. They were panicked that something serious was going on. I told them to go home, relax, and not start popping a damn pill. And for the obese, chain-smoking diabetics who wanted their youth back, I had something for them, too. I told them I had a remedy that required them taking it three times a week. Without risk of any side effects, it would lower their cholesterol, lower their blood pressure, lower their glucose levels, and potentially improve stamina and performance. They wanted it badly. When I explained to them the drug was called "exercise," they just moaned. They wanted a pill.

Aggressive advertising created this need for a quick fix. Never mind figuring out the cause for someone's erection problem, or formulating a long-term plan for treatment. Just prescribe and pop a pill.

I don't honestly believe this sequence of events was what the drug developers wanted or what the researchers intended. But the

CHAPTER 9 | *The Illness of Medicine*

marketing was ingenious, and I'm sure this group of drugs reached levels of sales light years beyond the original estimates. We also discovered that ours had become a quick-fix society. Take a downer at night, an upper in the day, a pill for sex. People wanted the easy, but not necessarily the right, treatment. And the price for the medications kept going up, because why not—the drug industry could get away with it. Treatment for a "disease" had indeed been identified. And now this "treatment" was really being abused, driving up demand and, with it, price.

The care and management of The Penis, particularly with regard to erections, became a field of specialization all its own. And it encompassed not just the physical aspect of erectile dysfunction but the entire psychology of what a penis is supposed to do.

We now have a new condition to manage, and the medical community can help with erectile dysfunction in a manner never even imagined just a generation ago. But among the considerations are not only how to treat the condition but whom to treat, when, and at what cost. Does the insurance company have an obligation to pay for this medication when the medication is generally being used for recreational purposes? Is the loss of an erection also affecting the psyche and well-being of the patient, and is insurance reimbursement therefore appropriate? How much medication (or coverage) is enough, and who should be able to make that determination? How does the loss of one's erection affect one's sexual partner, his or her needs and state of health?

Michael J. Young, M.D.

These are difficult questions that take the issue of erectile dysfunction to a different level of complexity. I don't presume to have definitive answers to these queries, but I want to point out that the medical understanding and treatment of this condition have introduced new variables, some of them subtle, that must be considered when prescribing or not prescribing these drugs.

These medications were a wonderful discovery. They had a role in our armamentarium for treating medical conditions, and they fulfilled a definite need—for the right patient. I prescribed them as necessary. My concern was that in our treatment of this condition, we also created a new one—a dependency on a pill. Little attempt was being made by many patients and their doctors to understand why the patients were having these erectile problems. Poor lifestyle choices that might have been the cause were simply overlooked, and were thereby tacitly condoned. It was easier for the doctor to prescribe a pill than to argue with a patient to change his bad habits.

My treatment plan was simple. Change your diet. Stop smoking. Lose weight. Cut down on the drinking. Take a vacation. Then let's talk and figure out the "why." Maybe then I'd prescribe a pill.

CHAPTER 10

Vasectomy

One of the most common procedures performed in urology is the vasectomy. Arguably, it is the most secure means of ensuring male sterility. A vasectomy involves cutting, cauterizing (burning), and based upon surgical technique, possibly removing a segment of the vas deferens, the tube that carries sperm from the epididymis (where sperm maturation and storage occur) and then it joins into the ejaculatory ducts. One of the reasons vasectomies are generally safe to perform is that the location of the tube can easily be determined by palpating (touching) the scrotum. Therefore, through a small, targeted incision in the scrotum, the urologist can access and operate on the vas deferens. Because the vas is so close to the skin in the scrotum, local anesthetic can be used. The procedure generally takes less than thirty minutes, and with an ice bag (or a bag of frozen peas) placed over the scrotum postoperatively, along with the use of mild analgesics, the vast majority of men do quite well. One of the most important things for the patient to understand before undergoing the procedure is that the vas deferens is a long structure, perhaps a foot or so in total length. The part of the structure that is most superficial, and

CHAPTER 10 | *The Illness of Medicine*

therefore most accessible to the urologist, is the initial segment located within the scrotum. This means that even after the tube is divided, the remaining ten inches or so of the vas deferens are still filled with sperm that are ready for ejaculation. In other words, there's still a possibility of causing pregnancy. All patients are informed that after the vasectomy, they are not to be considered sterile until a negative semen specimen is obtained, confirming that no sperm remain in the distal segment of the vas deferens. Generally, it takes around three months for all of the sperm beyond the area of division to be ejaculated out. During this time, the patients and their sexual partners must continue to use birth control until a negative semen specimen confirms sterility.

A very rare but possible complication of even a properly performed vasectomy is that the two cut ends of the vas deferens find their way back to each other. Obviously, this is an outcome that could result in a pregnancy. Again, this is very rare, but it is possible.

My practice was based in the near-north area of Chicago, which contains a mix of affluent professionals and blue-collar workers. The variety of the patients, their backgrounds influencing their understanding and management, always made the day interesting. In many ways, I found it very gratifying to be involved in the care of the less wealthy. They were generally kind people who worked very hard and were appreciative of their medical care. Some of the affluent, on the other hand, evinced a sense of entitlement and were a bit more challenging. Some, not all.

Michael J. Young, M.D.

One patient who was referred to me for a vasectomy was a producer for a television show. The reader can well imagine which of the aforementioned patient groups he represented. He was demanding, arrogant, and at best could be described as a jerk. Be that as it may, we had the customary preoperative discussion regarding expectations and risks and then, several weeks later, went ahead with the procedure.

His vasectomy went as well as the five hundred or so I'd already performed. The only deviation from the norm was the annoying frequency with which this patient called for additional postoperative pain medication. Eventually that died down as well, and the next conversation I had with the patient was regarding his post-vasectomy semen-specimen review. At that time, it was routine to obtain two separate specimens at three and four months out from the completion of the procedure, to confirm sterility. The more current guidelines mandate just one—if negative. He did the requisite semen analyses, both of them being without evidence of any sperm in the samples. He was happy. I was happy.

A year later I was the recipient of a most unpleasant phone call—a barrage of yelling, really. I was being threatened with a lawsuit by the patient who'd undergone the vasectomy. His girlfriend was now pregnant and, according to the patient, I was to blame.

There are few things more gut-wrenching than being threatened with a medical-malpractice claim. Despite the fact that the majority of suits don't progress beyond the threat phase, or are settled out of court, it is one of the most demoralizing, personally upsetting

CHAPTER 10 | *The Illness of Medicine*

events a physician can experience, and the legal process can grind on for years.

Although nothing legally had been filed by my former patient, his level of intensity, his absolute anger toward me, was palpable through the telephone. After hanging up the receiver, I went to his chart to reacquaint myself with the vasectomy of a man who was insinuating he would change my life forever. I looked through my notes: other than recalling what an entitled jerk he was, I saw nothing extraordinary in his records. The procedure was uneventful, and his postoperative semen studies were both negative. Certainly, recanalization (in this case, when the two cut ends of the vas deferens realign and become patent again) was a possibility, but my surgical technique was one of redundancy, designed to thoroughly minimize the risk of this happening. Upon making two separate scrotal incisions, I would always locate each vas deferens separately, and would ask the patient on which side he felt a pulling sensation to make certain I did not unwittingly repeat the procedure on the same side (leaving the other intact). I would resect (cut out) a reasonable length of the vas, and would then place a fine needle within the lumen (opening) of each side of the cut tube and apply electrocautery to seal each end. That alone would typically be enough, but I would then tie off the tip of each cut vas deferens with an absorbable suture, the goal being to induce a further degree of inflammation and scarring, and therefore closure. Finally, I would bury one end of the cut vas deferens under a layer of tissue, separate from the other, all to ensure that the two ends would not and could not migrate toward one another.

Michael J. Young, M.D.

(On the rare occasion that one of my patients desired a vasectomy reversal, technically referred to as a vasovasostomy, which involves reattaching the cut ends of the vas, I would dread having to undo my own work, knowing how much scar tissue there would be and the difficulty in the dissection.)

So, I was just devastated to think that my procedure/technique had failed despite all the precautions and effort taken to ensure it was done properly—well in excess of what was necessary to achieve the desired outcome. I called the patient back the next day and delicately explained to him the anatomy, and rare possibility, of recanalization. He appeared to listen intently to what I said. And then I suggested just one more thing—that he please submit another semen sample. Grudgingly, he said he would, protesting nonetheless that it would be a waste of time, given that his girlfriend was pregnant and no additional testing would change that outcome.

Four weeks later I received the lab results. His semen specimen was again negative. I was elated to know that despite his bullying threats to me, his insults and accusations, my surgical technique was still good. I called him up and—feeling a bit emboldened—informed him that I had good news and bad news. The good news was that he was sterile. The bad news was that he needed to find a new girlfriend. After a delay, I could hear a sigh. Did I go too far? Did my professional pride in knowing my procedure hadn't failed cause me to get a bit cocky? Or was I just happy as hell to know that this man in particular, who'd made my past four weeks absolute misery with his intimidation and threats, was wrong?

CHAPTER 10 | *The Illness of Medicine*

He spoke to me very quietly. I could barely hear his weakened voice on the telephone. Yes, he told me, he'd found out that his girlfriend was seeing someone else on the side. She was pregnant from another man. He hung up, without apology for the anguish he'd caused, without any consideration for what he'd put me through.

He had come in for a simple vasectomy. I did it, and I did it right. But when his girlfriend stepped out on him, he had to blame someone. I'm not surprised she strayed, but rather than consider the possibility that anyone could leave him, he went after his doctor from a year earlier.

I was relieved. But for what? I did a procedure for a patient who had requested it. I put my own reputation on the line doing what he'd asked me to do, and I did it properly. The legal pressure was off for the time being, but medicine is one of the few professions where the "client" can become a plaintiff against you even if you do your job right.

CHAPTER 11

The Fractured Testicle

Handling Friday-night call duty was always particularly stressful for me. Often it followed a busy week, and involved trying to avoid problems over the ensuing seventy-two hours while covering my practice and my partners'. If Friday night was bad, the weekend would almost certainly be difficult. Problems came in multiples—and tended to go from bad to worse.

One such weekend began on a beautifully clear, Chicago summer night. As usual for a call night, I went to bed around 10:00 p.m., hoping to get a reasonably good night's sleep. Often, that was difficult, not because of any specific call but because of the anticipation of the call. This particular weekend, my practice group was on emergency-room call, which meant that we were responsible for any "unassigned" patients, meaning those who presented to the ER without any prior patient-doctor relationship with a physician on staff. Many such patients had no insurance and had had limited if any previous medical care, and could therefore be the most challenging patients to take care of. There was no reference point

CHAPTER 11 | *The Illness of Medicine*

for the treating physician, and the patients were often suspicious of us and of "the system." Usually they were brought in by ambulance to the closest emergency room so that they could receive care from the specialists who were assigned that day or night.

On this night, I was awakened around 11:30 p.m. for a consultation regarding a testicular-trauma case. I could predict a long night ahead of me, along with a stressful remaining weekend, within ten seconds of hearing the reason for the interruption of my REM sleep. A forty-three-year-old man had suffered a fracture of the testicle.

The testicle is surprisingly resistant to injury, despite its exposed location, front and center, and also despite its being shielded by very little (scrotal skin is quite thin, and there's no significant layer of muscle or fat for protection). With a predilection for just hanging, the testicle would appear ripe for injury. But it is the very lack of resistance, the ability to be pushed aside in a compliant scrotal sac, that allows the testicle to avoid a significant injury when struck.

Most males who have gone through puberty have at one time or another felt the nauseating ache that comes with being hit firmly in the testicle. The pain, indescribably significant, causes one simply to bend over and drop to one's knees, barely able to utter a sound through the suffering. Embryologically, the testicle takes its origin in the vicinity of the kidneys, and throughout gestation (pregnancy) the testicle gradually moves into the scrotum during normal fetal development. The nerves and blood supply to the testicle have their origin up high in the posterior aspect of the abdomen. An injury to the testicle, from a sudden kick or blow, can consequently cause the pain to be experienced by the poor victim where the nerves originate. So with this type of injury, not only is there the local pain from the scrotum and testicle being struck but also the excruciating abdominal pain.

I walked into the ER around midnight and discovered, among other things, that the patient with the testicular fracture, who was lying on a gurney, was also articulate, educated, and insured. I had reviewed his scrotal ultrasound before examining him. The blow to the testicle had been so severe and sudden that the actual covering—the tough, fibrous shell around the testicular components (the seminiferous tubules responsible for sperm production, and the Leydig cells that produce testosterone)—was split open, causing the testicular contents to be expelled from inside the shell of the testicle. It was sort of like a cracked-open egg. You can only imagine the type of discomfort this would have caused at the moment of impact.

I examined the patient, confirming the diagnosis, and discussed with him the need for surgical exploration in an attempt to salvage the testicle, if possible. In some cases, the damage to a ruptured testicle is so severe that, without viable tissue to repair, the testicle needs to be removed.

Our conversation led to his revealing how the injury had occurred: He was hitting golf balls at a local driving range.

I am an avid golfer. I love the game—the history, the architecture of courses, the physics of how a ball flies. I often find myself daydreaming about playing a good round and how satisfying it feels to hit a golf ball solidly. The sound of the club striking the ball

CHAPTER 11 | *The Illness of Medicine*

properly is music to a golfer's ear. So how on earth did this golfer, hitting balls at a driving range, get here?

I knew the driving range quite well where he'd been practicing, as I'd hit balls there hundreds of times myself. It was a double-tiered range, curved to allow balls to be aimed toward the middle of the field. There were numerous light poles, for those of us who just can't get in enough practice during daylight hours. Apparently, the man practicing just to the right of the patient hit a nasty slice. When a right-handed golfer hits a slice, it means that the ball, when struck, spins in a fashion that makes it fly quickly to the right. Slices are common, the result of a swing error that every golfer commits now and again.

Unfortunately for the patient, the golfer with the vicious slice had decided to pull out his driver—the longest club in golfer's arsenal, and therefore the one used to hit the ball the hardest, and farthest. It was midday on a perfect summer afternoon. The man hit his ball so badly, with such force, and with such a terrible slice, that it ricocheted off a light pole (located right and slightly behind the golfers) and hit my patient smack in the scrotum.

The thought of the event—the sound of the impact, the pain involved—was dizzying. As I interviewed the patient prior to surgery, my heart sank that a fellow golf addict had suffered such injury while attempting to improve his swing. It was sad—a gentleman's game resulting in such trauma.

Michael J. Young, M.D.

But wait. According to my patient's story of woe, he'd been injured in the middle of the day, and it was now nearly midnight. I asked why it had taken him so long to present to the ER.

"I had to finish my bucket of balls," he replied.

I was unclear if I'd heard him properly. Had he really just said he pulled himself off the ground after suffering a testicular fracture and continued to hit balls? If so, I had a new hero!

He informed me that he'd limped back to his car after finishing his bucket of balls, driven home, and stretched out on the couch. Not until later, after doing a "Google search," had he learned that a "significant injury" might have occurred. He figured this must have explained the swelling and pain.

After hearing this, I wasn't so sure he was my hero anymore. If I had a scrotum that was starting to look like a pomegranate, and getting larger, I don't think I would be at home deciding whether to seek treatment.

I took him to surgery and was able to salvage the majority of the testicle. He did well, and went home the next day. My weekend was still in its infancy. Another day on call.

CHAPTER 12

Getting to the Office

How does a patient get to the doctor's office? I mean this in both the literal and figurative sense. It isn't as though a person can just walk into the front door of a private practice and expect to be seen and treated, right? Going to the doctor isn't like going to anything else—it is an event that has multiple layers and a defined protocol. So, let's look at the process.

First, something is wrong. This is not good. I know the feeling I have when my computer is on the fritz. I am anxious just knowing that not all is right and I need to get it repaired—it truly bothers me. It even keeps me up at night thinking about how the things I need to get done will be delayed until the repair is made. But my options are rather limited in this matter. Getting my computer fixed means resigning myself to endless hours on the telephone with someone named "Fred" from a country where they don't speak English. "Fred" and I will have a relationship that will start out fine. He is cordial. I am cordial. I don't understand most of what he says, but he sounds committed to helping me, so I tolerate his inability to communicate in English. I am, however, getting progressively

CHAPTER 12 | *The Illness of Medicine*

annoyed with how frequently "Fred" needs to put me on hold as he seeks out his supervisor (undoubtedly someone named "Ralph"). As the hours tick by, I start getting impatient with "Fred." My problem is not getting resolved, and now "Fred's" unintelligible English is starting to grind me down. We are quickly losing our rapport. I need to get this issue repaired, I need to get to bed, and I need it *now*. The original anxiety I experienced is quickly turning into anger. His unwavering calm is also getting to me. I need this resolved, and my own observance of courtesies has faded away. Does this series of events sound familiar? Well, I think it resembles the process of needing and seeking medical attention these days. Let's take a look.

Let's imagine an otherwise healthy forty-year-old male who wakes up one morning with a surprise. Let's give him a name: Jack. Jack goes to the washroom and notices that his urine is red. He feels no pain, and has no difficulty emptying his bladder. Jack really feels quite well. He goes through the mental process of reliving the past twenty-four hours. He tries to remember what he ate, and how much he had to drink. Maybe he just did too much exercise the day before. He decides to take a wait-and-see attitude, and the problem does in fact go away. The rest of the day is uneventful, and the rest of the week is fine. All is nearly forgotten, until it happens again. Interesting. Jack now does what nearly every "connected" patient does today: he goes online. He then realizes that the online information is at best vague and at worst telling him that he has two weeks to live. Jack finally admits he needs to see the doctor. Well, he hasn't seen his doc in years, but he'll pick up the phone and call to make an appointment—just to be safe.

Michael J. Young, M.D.

Jack must first go to his primary physician. He calls the office to set up an appointment. "Three weeks from tomorrow?" he asks. "That is all that is available? . . . Yes, I'll take it . . . No, I don't want to see his new associate. She's how old, and just graduated? . . . No, I'll wait, thank you. I don't think losing half a pint of blood each day in my urine should be an issue. I think I can make it. Do I have a choice?"

"Well, yes," the receptionist tells him. "You could always go to the emergency room." Most likely that would result in his undergoing a boatload of unnecessary tests, spending half the day there listening to someone moaning in the adjacent "room" (actually just a space on the other side of a paper-thin partition), and—after all that—being told to go see his personal doctor. He decides he can wait for the appointment. After all, he did see the blood a week or so previously and he's still okay.

Jack arrives at the office thirty minutes before his appointment time, as instructed. After filling out countless forms and reading every out-of-date *Guns & Ammo* magazine in the cramped, stuffy waiting room, he's summoned back into the working part of the office. Jack hasn't been to the doctor in years. He doesn't recall it ever being such a complicated, militarized process. The office staff act like automatons. It seems as if they really don't care. They probably don't.

He is called into the exam room. It has a funny smell—not just of rubbing alcohol but of something else besides. Maybe it's a mixture of cleaning solution, some bodily fluid like urine, and just old worn-

CHAPTER 12 | *The Illness of Medicine*

out carpeting. The nurse who brought him into the room seems to be lacking anything remotely like a smile. Jack thinks she has the personality of cardboard and that she's best suited for working in a cemetery.

He waits in the six-foot-by-six-foot exam room for what seems like an eternity. The walls of the room must be made of construction paper, as he can hear everything going on in the hallway and in the adjacent room. He listens to the laughter in one room, the crying in the next. The telephone in the hallway seems to be ringing constantly. Quiet and calm, it isn't. Finally, the doctor comes in. Jack remembers him being a nice enough fellow. But the doc appears different than Jack recalled. He now appears rushed, a bit discombobulated. During the perfunctory handshake, Jack notices that the doctor's hands are damp—maybe he just washed them? Gone is the time when they chatted a bit before getting down to business. Now it is *all* business. "So, what's the problem?" the doctor asks. Jack explains why he's there, but the doctor never really looks at him, preoccupied instead with typing away at his computer. He occasionally makes a grunting noise, not because of the medical problem but because he's made errors while typing. The physician has the same glazed appearance of pseudo-concern that the nurse had. The doc agrees, however, that blood in the urine isn't a good thing. That's reassuring, Jack thinks. The doctor has him give a urine sample. It's red. "There is blood in it," the doctor explains helpfully. Jack takes a blood test. The doctor rechecks Jack's vital signs. Jack surmises that he isn't going to keel over that day. The doctor gives him a referral to a urologist.

Michael J. Young, M.D.

A *referral*—the golden ticket to being cured. The document states that it will expire ninety days after being tendered. Jack is told to go see the specialist in that time frame. Like he's going to wait? It's already been nearly a month. What a system. How did being a patient become so difficult? When did the primary physician become a de facto clerical worker—one who spends more time documenting information and giving out referrals than actually treating patients?

Now let's change the scenario. We have an elderly woman as the patient. She's somewhat frail, has difficulty hearing, and is certainly unable to drive herself. She too has blood in her urine. Her daughter calls the primary office for an appointment. The diligent daughter must take time off from work to be able to assist her mother. Parking is a problem. Medical centers have become so large, so sprawling, that simply negotiating the distance from the parking lot to the medical office building can routinely take a half an hour—and our patient doesn't move that well. Her daughter needs to get a wheelchair. Where are they? There is no help to be found. With some good luck, an abandoned wheelchair is located near the exit. Is there ever a wheelchair that actually has four working wheels? And why do they always seem to want to drift to one side or the other, never rolling straight? What is that clicking noise the wheelchair makes as it barely moves despite the considerable force being exerted to push it? With the one-hour trek on the expressway, navigating through the construction-zone traffic, and now parking and getting into the wheelchair, the process is just exhausting. Onward to the doctor's office.

CHAPTER 12 | *The Illness of Medicine*

The elevator is slow, but finally they arrive at the office. Opening the heavy glass door while moving the wheelchair out of the way, and then getting through before the door closes, is difficult. The move would rate a seven out of ten in Olympic gymnastics. The patient's daughter is worn out. They wait in the musty waiting room. The receptionist has a bit of an attitude given that they were thirty minutes late for their appointment. Seriously? And *forms*. More forms to fill out than for a mortgage. Does anybody really read what is filled out? All of the office staff keep asking the same questions.

As the patient is wheeled into the exam room, the damn chair will not easily get through the doorway. Isn't there some Americans with Disabilities Act mandate regarding the size of doorways? Got to make sure Mother doesn't lose a leg or foot while squeezing the wheelchair through the narrow entrance. Another challenge for an already difficult day, just to be seen by the primary physician. As in our previous patient's appointment, the physician comes in a bit frazzled. A cursory, seemingly meaningless exam is performed—so little time. Got to keep up the quota. Remember, only fifteen minutes allowed per patient. Again, missing is the "human touch" of yore. There are no pleasantries. There *is* more typing into the computer. Eye contact? That is really asking too much.

When our elderly patient is wheeled back through the maze of the office, she and her daughter have to check out with the receptionist. There's the damn copay. Sort of like having to pay baggage fees on the airline. Shouldn't the copay just be included in the exorbitant insurance premium in the first place?

Unfortunately, the patients described are the lucky ones. Some make the effort and in the end are seen only by the nurse. But not to worry (the latter patients are assured), the nurse is experienced (two years out of training) and will certainly review "every detail" with the doctor. Promise. The doctor will call if there are any questions. Unlikely.

But if nothing else, a referral is generated. All that time, all that energy, all the scheduling and inconvenience, etc., are just a means of obtaining a voucher for actual medical attention at the *next* appointment. Welcome to the world of American medical care, 2018. No actual care is provided, but another step is checked off on a long list of what needs to be done in order to receive eventual treatment.

So our two patients have now marked off step one in the process of getting care: Forget that even though they saw their primary physician, little of actual medical consequence occurred. Forget that they took an entire day off from work and made alternate plans. The most important thing is that they got their boarding pass to see the specialist. The buck has now been passed. The primary has done his job. He typed some mumbo jumbo into the electronic medical-record system and out popped the referral to the specialist. One hopes that he did a thorough evaluation and properly checked other aspects of the patient's status to ensure that other medical issues weren't looming.

Of course, it should be noted that the patients did have another option. Rather than enduring the rigmarole of going through the

CHAPTER 12 | *The Illness of Medicine*

standard primary M.D. process, some patients (most often a bit wealthier) will have a *concierge* physician. Those lucky few who do will pay up front for the opportunity to have their primary M.D. tend to their needs. Often, they will pay at least several thousand dollars a year to the primary physician. That primary, as a consequence of having entered into this arrangement, will typically limit his or her practice to a select number of patients. For those patients, however, attention is significantly improved. They can call their physicians more directly and have much more efficient evaluations. They don't need to pay separate baggage fees and can board the plane early. Of course, they too paid their fees—it's just not as obvious and itemized.

Getting to see a specialist is not necessarily an easy task. Once the referral is generated, simply getting an appointment can still take weeks, sometimes months. Unfortunately, problems don't always wait that long before getting worse. But for those fortunate enough to avoid a trip to the ER, seeing the specialist might be just another round among many in finding "the cure."

Both of our patients will be seen. Typically, some form of imaging (e.g., x-rays) will be ordered by the specialist, as well as blood tests or other preoperative evaluations. And this can mean a return to the primary's office for the necessary referrals if the specialist doesn't have either the facilities for such tests or the authorization to write referrals for them. By now our patients and their families are getting away from the "frightened" phase of disease and entering the "frustration" phase. Recall the computer-repair analogy we started with. The honeymoon is over, the problem continues, and the bureaucracy of getting evaluation and treatment is pilling on. Our patients didn't see this in the fancy brochure the insurance company sent to them once they paid their first premium. The brochure features a healthy family on its cover. Everybody is smiling in the brochure photograph. Nice white teeth. The photograph is taken in a park or on a swing set in a nice backyard. There are no wheelchairs in the picture.

The patients get their tests. A procedure of some form is also indicated. The blood in the patients' urine mandates a look into the bladder, possibly a look into the kidneys. Another round of referrals is necessary, but fortunately this level of referrals can usually be obtained through the specialist's office. But the patients have to go back to their primary physician anyway for the "preoperative history and physical." This is an evaluation required to ensure that the patients are healthy enough to undergo the procedure dictated by their medical condition. The reevaluation is necessary because more than a month has passed since the problems were first seen by the primary physicians, and anesthesia regulations require that patients be seen by their primary within thirty days of an upcoming procedure. The "frustration" phase of illness is now in full gear. But this is just the beginning. Our patients have yet to deal with the hospital and its extraordinarily inefficient processes.

Anywhere from twelve to twenty-four months later, our patients will receive a bill from the hospital for services provided. The document will undoubtedly be written in a form of hieroglyphics that only an advanced medical biller could understand. Not only will that invoice be uninterpretable, but more than likely, the

CHAPTER 12 | *The Illness of Medicine*

explanation of what was actually performed, what warranted that bill in the first place, will be so cryptic that even the most astute patient will not understand the what, when, and how of it all. Next, reams of paperwork from the insurance company delineating what it will and will not cover will show up in the mail. Confusing? Just a tad. The billing and payment process alone will induce an ulcer and a migraine headache of such proportions that more medical attention will be warranted.

And for all the effort to this point, neither patient has yet received treatment! Somehow, in this mess of a system, the medical community has lost sight of the realization that a person, not just "another patient," has a medical problem in need of treatment.

And so, the inefficient wheels of the medical world turn. This process is repeated over and over in doctors' offices all across the country.

Fear, frustration, and eventually anger.

I believe these emotions describe the experience today of having a medical problem, and how the process of seeking treatment and help is compromised. Being sick is difficult enough. But how patients are *managed*—the lack of empathy, the effort and energy required to navigate through a complex system—can be absolutely infuriating. But what choices do the patients really have? They just want to get better and move on with their lives.

CHAPTER 13

So, You Need Surgery

The very thought of needing surgery is troubling. It means that something inside of our body, something we can't otherwise control, is broken. Something within is not functioning properly, and there is no elixir, pill, diet, or activity to fix it. I was once told during my second year of medical school that there are basically three reasons for pathology—for things not to be right within our body:

The parts are bad.

The parts are worn out.

You have no luck.

We all want to be healthy. Everything else in our lives diminishes in importance when our physical well-being is in jeopardy. Health is our most precious commodity.

Obviously, we would prefer the least toxic, least intrusive, and most effective means of mitigating or improving what is not functioning properly. Be it a clogged vessel, a painful hip, a

CHAPTER 13 | *The Illness of Medicine*

congenital abnormality, an injury—when something mechanical fails to respond to conservative treatment, or there is no other alternative care, our only remaining option is to physically go in and make adjustments.

In facing the majority of medical problems, I am a strong advocate for the most effective, most tested of treatments: time. But time will not remove the blood clot from the brain, or dissolve the tumor that is growing. When I was still practicing, surgery was my last option for most diseases. To cut is not always to cure. Sometimes to cut is just to cut. I sincerely believe that the hardest part of surgery for the physician is not the actual surgery itself. The most difficult part—as it should be, and must be—is deciding whether surgery is necessary. On the other end of the knife is a person—a mother, sister, brother. Sometimes bad things can happen inadvertently with a scalpel, and such risks are not to be undertaken casually.

I taught young resident surgeons for years about what Woody Hayes, the former Ohio State football coach, supposedly said about passing the football: "When you throw a football into the air," said Hayes, "three things can happen, two of which are bad." The ball can be dropped or intercepted. The odds for the desired outcome, that the ball is caught by the intended receiver, can be long, though the reward can be great in the event of success. Surgery can be the same.

I was once consulted to see an eighty-five-year-old patient of mine who was in the hospital. Twenty years earlier, after a cancer diagnosis, I'd taken out his prostate, and the day before this current visit he'd had a "simple" (outpatient) hernia repair, performed by another surgeon. The repair, however, had taken much longer than expected. From a urological standpoint, he'd been stable prior to the recent surgery, but postoperatively he had developed urinary retention (he couldn't urinate), so a Foley catheter needed to be placed into his bladder. The need for this is not uncommon after long surgery, particularly in the elderly.

But he'd been anticipating a relatively quick hernia procedure, having been told that it would take "about an hour or so." Why, then, had his outpatient procedure taken so much longer than anticipated? Why had it resulted in—or at least coincided with—urinary retention and the need for a catheter? This was not clear to me. What *was* clear was that he was not doing well. Furthermore, I knew the reputation of his surgeon, and it involved a higher than expected number of surgical complications.

The patient's abdomen was distended, meaning that it was enlarged. This is typically because of gas in the intestinal tract. Patients young or old can have gas collect in the intestines from the effects of anesthesia, analgesia (pain medication), or lack of activity. In essence, the intestines were not propelling their contents in the normal, peristaltic manner. But this was excessive, particularly since his surgery had occurred only a day prior to my seeing him. When I arrived in his room he was eating. Why, I wondered, had a meal been served to him when his abdomen was so enlarged? His intestinal tract needed to rest—to be spared the effort of digesting the French toast he was shoveling down. I asked his nurse why he was being served a full meal given his current status. She didn't know, but said she was "following orders." I contacted the general

CHAPTER 13 | *The Illness of Medicine*

surgical resident that was assigned to him, who assured me he would visit the patient.

The following day, I entered the patient's room to find him now with a nasogastric tube in place. This is a tube that is passed through the patient's nose into his stomach to decompress the gastrointestinal tract—literally, to suck the gas out. This is a miserable tube to have inserted. As uncomfortable as the catheter in the penis may appear, patients complain of this tube even more. His belly was still enlarged. He went for additional x-rays and was found to have such an extreme amount of gas in his intestinal tract that the cecum (the very beginning of the large intestine) was dangerously dilated. He was now being scheduled to have it decompressed from the other end by a gastroenterologist using a colonoscope.

During the subsequent procedure, the gastroenterologist couldn't pass the instrument up to the specific point. Then the cecum blew out. Intestinal gas was now outside of the colon and within the abdominal cavity. This is a true emergency.

The patient went back to surgery immediately and underwent a colon resection. A segment of his colon had to be removed. Given the significant abdominal infection that had occurred from the bowel perforation, he was subsequently admitted to the surgical intensive care unit, where he resided for over a month.

The patient eventually recovered. He lost forty pounds, and upon leaving the ICU he had to stay in the hospital another month for rehabilitation. But finally he was discharged, and free of the Foley catheter. All that for a simple outpatient hernia repair.

Michael J. Young, M.D.

There is no such thing as "simple" surgery. There is only surgery. And again, in the words of Woody Hayes, three things can happen, and two of them are bad. Actually, in surgery there are literally hundreds of things that can happen, but there's only one desirable outcome—an uneventful recovery.

To cut is not necessarily to cure. Surgery should be utilized only when there is no other reasonable treatment available. Period.

* * * * * * * * * *

So, you need surgery? Okay, fine. Do your homework. By that I do not mean spend hours on the internet trying to learn the procedure. Essentially, your surgeon has already done that for you. It is time, however, for you to learn about the surgeon himself or herself. Ask how many times he or she has performed the procedure you need. What is the surgeon's expected usual time of recovery? What is the frequency of complications? Obtain a second opinion as a matter of course, not because you might think your surgeon is wrong but to verify whether an alternative intervention, or even alternative procedures, may be applied to your particular medical condition. Again, obtain a second opinion.

For example, we are now in an era of surgery in which many procedures can be performed either via an "open" technique (meaning, through an incision) or laparoscopically (performed through multiple pen-sized openings). The advantage of the open

CHAPTER 13 | *The Illness of Medicine*

procedure is that the surgeon has nearly complete access to the structures he is operating on. It is considered the "gold standard" with regard to surgical control. Up until the last thirty years, this was effectively the only way for many surgeries to be performed. However, many procedures can now be performed utilizing multiple small laparoscopic instruments. The advantage is that having smaller access "ports" allows for a significantly faster recovery. There is no major incision, and therefore much less incidental tissue damage to heal. Consequently, there is less pain and an earlier return to activities following a laparoscopic procedure. There may also be a technical advantage in the laparoscopic approach, such as optical magnification and better visualization. The risk, however, is that the surgeon, working through much smaller instruments, has potentially less control should problems arise. The surgeon is also relying almost solely on visual technique, with limited tactile sensation during the procedure. The surgeon may also be unable to complete the procedure for technical reasons.

We are in an era in surgery when there are still many (slightly older) surgeons trained only in the standard open techniques. Conversely, some younger surgeons may have only limited experience in the open approach. I think it would be reasonable to seek opinions from surgeons regarding both approaches before committing to one or the other.

I highly recommend a discussion with one's family or supporting individuals before undergoing any major procedure. Many patients come into the office for a problem that requires surgery, but they fail to appreciate what happens *after* the procedure. Some patients decide to keep the issue to themselves, even though they will likely need help with the basics of daily living. Bear in mind that no matter how "minor" the procedure may seem to the surgeon—as he or she may have performed it possibly hundreds of times—that same surgeon has probably never been the patient undergoing the procedure. With postoperative pain or limited mobility, the patient might discover that the usually simple tasks of shopping for groceries, walking up and down stairs, even getting in and out of a bed or a shower, can be extraordinarily difficult until the recovery has progressed. Driving will often not be allowed in the immediate postoperative period, and as a postoperative visit for dressing changes or other follow-up may be necessary, one will need to arrange help getting to and from the doctor's office. I think an honest evaluation of one's postoperative requirements must be made prior to the surgery date, and that friends or family must be alerted to their potential need to help. Nothing will alienate friends more quickly than an "emergency" imposition that could actually have been anticipated and planned for, had they only been given some advance notice.

* * * * * * * * * *

Before any surgery can be performed in most hospitals today, patients must be "cleared" for the procedure by either their primary physician or a preadmission testing clinic. These clinics are often run by hospital anesthesia departments. Patients need to be

CHAPTER 13 | *The Illness of Medicine*

evaluated to see if they are able to undergo anesthesia safely. This requires basic blood testing, possible x-rays, and possibly an EKG (electrocardiogram). If a patient has a history of previous cardiac or pulmonary (lung) conditions, a cardiology evaluation, including a possible cardiac stress test, may be required.

As a surgeon, I can tell you that one of the most frequent reasons for a surgical case to be canceled is the use of anticoagulants (blood thinners)—or, more often than not, the patient's forgetting to stop taking the anticoagulants in the days leading up to surgery. These medicines are now being prescribed so frequently that I rarely saw a patient over the age of seventy-five who was not on one of the many drugs available to thin one's blood. They are often prescribed to inhibit blood-clot formation, clots being of particular concern if one has an artificial heart valve, a coronary stent, or a history of peripheral vascular disease or stroke. But they inhibit clotting so well that it is a problem for surgeons, who need bleeding to stop on its own. Many patients who aren't on prescribed anticoagulants are nonetheless on a daily aspirin regimen—regular or low dose. This medication effects platelet function, thereby impeding blood-clot formation, and therefore it must also be discontinued a week prior to the surgery, unless the patient is directed otherwise.

Alcohol is another "drug" that is often overlooked by patients prior to surgery. In addition to its other known properties, alcohol, too, can promote bleeding. There is nothing more frustrating than to have a patient go through the whole process of preoperative preparation—family and friends waiting, follow-up management arranged—and then to realize as he or she is sitting in the preoperative holding area that surgery must be delayed because it turns out the patient had had a "few" drinks the night before. In many cases, this will cause the train to stop in its tracks. Everyone will be upset, including the surgeon, who has allotted a portion of the day for your procedure. Stop the beer, the wine, and the cocktails at least seven days prior to your procedure (unless instructed otherwise). And since all patients will do better with clear lungs, stop the smoking, too.

* * * * * * * * * *

The day has come for surgery. Plan on arriving at the hospital two hours prior to scheduled surgery time, but be prepared to wait. Surgery scheduling is much like managing an airline fleet today: your plane can't take off until the incoming flight has arrived and been unloaded, cleaned, checked, and refueled. If the surgical case in the operating room ahead of you has delays or unforeseen issues that mandate additional time, your operation will consequently be later than scheduled. Realize you have the day off and just roll with it. Pestering the staff isn't really an option. Calm is good.

Change into a hospital gown designed by someone who has never had to wear one. Understand that putting on the idiotically designed gown and not having your derriere exposed is just not possible, so accept it and move on. Keeping one's vanity in a hospital setting is simply not possible. Nobody really cares, as the hospital staff has seen everything anyway.

CHAPTER 13 | *The Illness of Medicine*

Go along with what the nurses tell you to do. If you make their lives easier, the nurses undoubtedly will be grateful and kind in return. Remember, they really have probably seen it all, and they don't need an imperious patient pushing their buttons.

An IV (intravenous line for fluid and drug access) will be placed in your arm or hand. The same questions will be asked of you multiple times, by multiple people. Refrain from pointing this out to them. Everyone in the surgical section is trying to do the right thing to ensure your safety. They are verifying, for instance, that you *do not* have a specific allergy or that you *have* properly stopped whatever medication you were supposed to stop. The preoperative personnel are ensuring that the right procedure is being done on the right patient. Be tolerant and cooperative as they go through their checklists. Do not forget that the nursing personnel may have ten to fifteen patients *that same day* undergoing the same procedure as you. Whether it's having a cataract removed, a hernia repaired, or a hip or knee replaced, the nurses must confirm that the right patient is having the designated procedure—and on the correct side. Any mistake that could have been prevented is not acceptable. Preoperative questioning and requestioning and operative site marking must be performed.

The preoperative wait can feel like an eternity. You are undoubtedly hungry, as part of the preoperative process requires that you not eat or drink for a minimum of six to eight hours prior to surgery. This is done as a precautionary measure related to anesthesia. Should any regurgitation (vomiting) occur during the induction of anesthesia, the medical staff does not want to risk having you aspirate any vomit into your lungs. Better to have an empty stomach and be hungry for a few hours than have to recover from a potentially life-threatening pulmonary injury.

Despite all possible appearance to the contrary, however, progress is being made toward getting you into surgery. However . . .

* * * * * * * * * *

One of my significant complaints about hospital surgical departments was a consistent failure to organize people. A hospital may have had the most-sophisticated surgical instrumentation, a famous surgeon, and a staff of dedicated individuals ready to perform that unique surgical procedure. But for reasons that simply did not make sense to me, getting from point A (walking through the door of the hospital surgical department) to point B (being delivered on a gurney to the operative suite) appeared to resemble Brownian motion. Brownian motion is a physical chemistry kinetic theory describing the random movement of particles suspended in a fluid. In other words, things just ran into one another until, as a consequence of chance, actual progression occurred. And yes, I understand the complexity of what is always going on in surgical departments:

The patient must check in.

The patient must change clothes.

CHAPTER 13 | *The Illness of Medicine*

Verification must be performed and history checked.

The patient must be seen by anesthesia and have an IV started.

The patient must see the surgeon, consent to surgery, and have the site of surgery marked and reverified.

The operative suite must be turned over (cleaned from the previous case).

The new operative team must prepare the room and have the necessary equipment made ready and then counted. (The instruments, sponges, and suture needles must be counted both before and after the procedure to ensure that nothing was left in the patient. Although this may seem an almost ridiculous precaution, in long procedures with multiple nurses, assistants, and possibly surgeons, or in procedures involving large wounds, things can potentially get left behind.)

The patient must be brought into the operative suite.

But why this sequence of events wasn't better coordinated was beyond my comprehension. Often, I found myself actually calling the operating-room manager and informing him or her that:

I am ready.

The patient is ready.

The room is ready—let's go!

Typically, I had to make a trip to where the anesthesiologists hung out in order to grab one. I needed to push the system.

Such poor coordination is not a problem encountered at most outpatient surgical centers. They are usually geared for less complex cases and more regularly perform the same procedure over and over. However, there is also a financial incentive at these centers to get the cases completed. Possibly there is a bonus for the employees to be efficient.

* * * * * * * * * *

So, you are finally on your way to surgery. The family has said their goodbyes, and you have been placed onto the transportation gurney. A blanket that feels as thin as paper is placed over you. If the operative suites and preoperative holding areas are not on the same floor, you are moved into an elevator.

I've probably been in tens of thousands of elevators in my life. They go up; they go down. Some move quickly, and most move slower than desired. But riding in elevators with patients about to go to surgery reveals just how vulnerable patients can feel. One can see it in their faces. They are transported in the most defenseless position: lying down, with a stranger at the head of the gurney who is pushing. Most likely the orderly has bumped the gurney into the walls of the elevator several times. While enduring these collisions the patients are probably wondering if this orderly has had his driver's license revoked. Of course, the elevator space is much too small for the task at hand. And despite the "transport only" sign outside of the

CHAPTER 13 | *The Illness of Medicine*

dedicated elevator entrance, others are on the elevator as well. Who bothers reading signage? Conversations continue above the patients lying there. The patients are wearing a gown that most likely has not been tied closed because it would take an advanced design degree to figure that maneuver out. Of course, there's the paper-thin sheet too. Any wonder why the patients might feel that all on-board are gazing upon them in their near-naked exposure? Maybe it's because the others on the cramped elevator are doing just that. The patients have an IV in their arm that is uncomfortable, and they are hungry. It's early morning, and the additional riders on the elevator have their coffees—and continue to slurp loudly.

But what is most obvious on the faces of patients as they arrive in the preoperative holding area is their awareness that *they are not in control*. Among the many thoughts racing through patients' heads at this time is the fact that they have signed multiple legal authorization forms in the previous area, none of which made any sense. Most people have an attorney present to review paperwork when signing for work issues or a mortgage. Yet in this environment—one of potential life or death—they sign the papers quickly and without really reading any of the small print. Who has the time or is in the proper frame of mind at this particular moment? Multiple times patients are warned in the documents that complications or even death can occur from the procedure they are about to undergo. As a surgeon quite familiar with those forms, even I didn't really understand what usable information they were conveying to patients—other than that they might not make it out alive. The patients sign the forms anyway. I think it would make more sense legally (for both hospitals and patients) as well as emotionally (for patients), if the patients were given the paperwork days ahead of time for review. As part of any such "legal" agreement, signatories should have the time to actually read, consider, and understand what they are putting their names to.

Emerging from the elevator, patients are carted away by a stranger to an unfamiliar place. They feel almost bare, and the temperature appears to be near freezing. Given that the surgeon and operating staff are always wearing two layers of covering (their scrub clothes and a sterile gown over that) plus a cap, a mask, and one or two layers of gloves, they can get quite warm, particularly under the bright lights of the operating room. This explains why the room temperature is kept so cool. Interestingly, under general anesthesia patients are effectively paralyzed, and their normal thermoregulatory mechanisms are effected. Hypothermia is actually possible. Current anesthesia regulations require that body temperature be monitored and stabilized. If a patient's temperature drops too low at any point, significant medical consequences could occur.

Again, after waiting what probably feels like an eternity, patients are then brought into the operating room. I suspect that for the average, mentally balanced, well-nourished, moderately healthy (if possibly a tad overweight) person reading this description, this process probably doesn't sound too remarkable. However, for someone who is ill, injured, scared, young, or elderly, this can be quite a daunting experience. Many very good nurses do their best

CHAPTER 13 | *The Illness of Medicine*

to ease the patients' tension. But with a mask covering their facial expressions, even nurses who smile look intimidating.

* * * * * * * * * *

You are transferred onto the operating-room table. You either move under your own power—of course being careful not to expose yourself—or you are lifted by the staff. Two things are immediately evident to you: The table is hard, and the table is narrow. Remember, this isn't the Hyatt, and it's a table you're on, not a comfortable, down-filled mattress. The bright lights are moved into position. As the anesthesiologist looms over you, he is behind your head—I can imagine that everything looks upside down. You will possibly now hear the operating team go over the upcoming case (you!) out loud. This is another safety measure to help ensure that the right patient is undergoing the right procedure on the proper side. An inventory is taken of any unusual equipment requested by the surgeon, to verify that such equipment is in the room and ready to be used.

This is the theory, at least. There were times I was in the OR waiting to start a case and only then discovered that although the equipment was present and available, nobody had bothered to test it. It's a terrible feeling when after all this preparation and effort have been expended, you try to turn on the laser device and realize too late that it's not working. More than a few expletives are shouted out at such times.

Michael J. Young, M.D.

Rule #1 to OR personnel: Please test the equipment prior to the scheduled case.

Rule #2 in the OR: It is always good practice to have a calm anesthesiologist. Nothing scares a patient more than hearing an anesthesiologist—the person about to take control of the patient's vital functions (breathing, heart rate, blood pressure, temperature)—screaming at his residents or staff.

If and when everything is under control, the anesthesiologist will inject medicine into the IV. It will burn a bit, but it won't last but a few seconds. Think of all the steps it took to get to this point: the initial diagnosis in the office, the follow-up x-rays and lab tests, the repeated discussions with the physician, the preoperative evaluation, and the procedures in the hospital just prior to the actual surgery. Think of the time and energy—the wasted energy—spent getting referrals for each step. Think of all of the emotional drain, the late-night conversations you had with yourself and your family or loved ones. A lot of blood, sweat, and tears (literally) went into the decision to proceed. And suddenly it will all go black.

A breathing tube might then be placed into your mouth or down into your windpipe (trachea), depending on the type of procedure and if paralysis is necessary. For some procedures, epidural anesthesia is administered. In these cases, the numbing medication is injected into your spine to anesthetize a particular area, allowing you to remain conscious during the surgery. The decision to utilize this type of anesthesia is based on the bodily location of the surgery, the length of time anticipated for the procedure, and

CHAPTER 13 | *The Illness of Medicine*

the patient's health and postoperative recovery expectations. For some conditions, doctors need the epidural to provide pain relief for several days postoperatively. In particular cases, the patient may be immobilized during that time, and this is a desirable anesthetic choice.

* * * * * * * * *

After anesthetic is administered in the OR, the patient is now asleep. *In a drug-induced reversible coma* is probably a more accurate description. The operating-room staff will now "prep and drape," meaning they will prepare the operative site—shaving it, washing it with a disinfectant, and placing towels and draping sheets over it to isolate the operative field/region. The surgeons now "scrub." I'm sure most readers are familiar with surgeons on television disinfecting their hands and arms with a scrubbing solution prior to putting on their sterile gloves. Today, however, scrubbing is most often performed by placing a highly concentrated, quickly evaporating, alcohol-based or other chemical disinfectant on the surgeon's hands and arms. This is somewhat similar to what people do almost everywhere in our current germophobic society. The solution used in the operating rooms, however, is applied with greater care and consistency and is very potent. (I'm convinced that having applied this harsh chemical to my own hands and arms for years, I'm fated to experience something very bad years from now. I doubt that lab rats, through threat or reward, could ever be conditioned to rub this stuff on their little paws day after day for years, yet I did it all the time of my own free will.)

If this were a movie, we'd now come to the scene where the surgeons burst into the operating room with their scrubbed hands raised in the air. In reality, surgeons usually just walk into the room with hands elevated, careful not to touch anything—water is no longer running down their forearms onto the floor. The scrub nurse (the nurse who is assisting with the procedure, passing instruments, etc.) will then hand the surgeon a gown that is tied behind by a non-sterile nurse. (Referred to as the circulator, the non-sterile nurse circulates in and out of the room during the procedure to obtain necessary equipment, to document events during the procedure, etc.) Gloves are placed over the surgeon's hands by the scrub nurse. Final draping is placed over the patient, and another "time-out" is called to review the patient's name and procedure and to verify that the correct "side" of the patient is about to be operated on, and then, finally, the procedure actually begins. The scalpel is applied.

I honestly believe the hardest part of performing the surgery is the *decision* to perform the surgery. With time, practice, and proper mentoring, most surgical residents will learn to operate. Through years of observation, and then of gradual engagement in doing more and more of each procedure, most students will become proficient in the operation they are studying and intending to master. They will learn where to place their hands and when to look for this or that particular structure or organ. They will learn not just the maneuvers but the proper *sequencing* of maneuvers involved in safely removing, reconstructing, or destroying whatever it is they're

CHAPTER 13 | *The Illness of Medicine*

targeting in a given procedure. They will make their incision, do their work, and then close things up. But what cannot easily be taught is the *judgment* behind knowing when, or even if, to do the surgery.

I was trained to remove a cancerous prostate gland, using both open and robotic procedures. I could do it and do it well. The most difficult part of the equation was deciding on which patient—with how much disease, with what concomitant medical problems, with what life expectancy, etc.—to perform the procedure. Any such procedure will essentially be a technical repeat each time, with perhaps some individual modifications. The surgeon spends years learning how to do the steps consistently and—most important— to end up with *consistent results*. But teaching judgment to the person wielding the knife is a more elusive process. How does an art professor teach a student how to paint? He simply can't. The professor can teach technique, suggest alternative materials, possibly give the art student a historical background regarding an issue. But the student either has the eye, the intuition, and the desire to express himself or he doesn't. Perhaps the same can be said of teaching surgery. The student either has it or he doesn't.

I observed junior residents who demonstrated outstanding hand-eye coordination, smoothly performing procedures that certain more-senior residents were performing with wasted steps and less finesse. The senior residents went on to graduate, but they likely never acquired the same proficiency. I could have worked hard to demonstrate to the senior residents more-elegant techniques to improve their skill sets. But the residents were either able to incorporate the skills or not, and more teaching wasn't going to give them more dexterity or subtlety in a complex maneuver. Yet they were still qualified to graduate and perform the operation.

As the knife is applied, do you really know which class of student is now operating on you? Obviously not. You interviewed your surgeon, and you were most likely referred to him or her by your primary, whom you trust. But it's actually hard to know in advance if your surgeon has "good hands."

I have seen some surgeons better suited to carpentry than to surgery. I say that tongue-in-cheek. These surgeons have fulfilled educational qualifications, and although their outcomes are satisfactory, they could be a good degree better. Their incisions are larger than everyone else's. Their procedures somehow always take longer and end up being "more difficult" than anticipated. Their patients' recovery times and postoperative pain levels always appear far worse than others'. So why do patients go to them? Because the patients trust them. These surgeons communicate well with their patients and have good bedside rapport with them. So, despite the ham-handedness, they have earned their patients' confidence and are now performing surgery on them.

* * * * * * * * * *

So the procedure continues, with whatever degree of finesse. Some thoughts on procedures:

CHAPTER 13 | *The Illness of Medicine*

I feel that if the surgery to be performed is rather straightforward and the surgeon to perform it has a well-documented history of good outcomes, it can be performed at either a community hospital or a university center. One difference between the two is that at the former, the patient is more likely to have his surgery performed by the surgeon he is scheduled with. In a university setting, although the attending surgeon will be present throughout the procedure (or at least critical portions of it), the surgery will more likely be handled by a surgical resident or fellow (a physician who has already completed his/her residency and is now learning subspecialized training). This is all part of the teaching process. This is how the art and science of surgery has been passed on since the very first operation was performed. All senior attending surgeons were students at one time.

If a patient has a rather unique problem requiring the skills of a more specially trained surgeon, or a problem whose treatment mandates complex integration of multiple medical services, the university setting is appropriate. Some patients prefer being in the university regardless of the complexity of their medical condition. Others prefer the privacy and generally more direct interaction with their own doctor in the community hospital. In general, community hospitals are smaller and more efficient than tertiary university hospitals. The primary determinant of where to go for treatment should be the medical issue itself. You simply want to know that the facility is well suited to treating your problem. Everything else is of vanishing importance. The hospital is not a hotel. You're not planning to reside there as a guest. You shouldn't be focusing on amenities that aren't vital to your surgical outcome. You are there to get your treatment and, literally, get the hell out (as directed by your insurance company).

In general, the operating room is quite busy during a case. The anesthesiologist, sitting at the head of the table, is constantly monitoring the patient's status. The surgeon and his assistants are performing their case, often with intense focus.

There are moments of complete silence, as when a particularly detailed maneuver is being performed. During such complex or difficult steps, absolute concentration is required. But during the bulk of most procedures, certainly during the more repetitive sections of surgery (opening, setting retractors, closing), discussions are common and can vary widely, touching on everything from routine life events to interesting social plans. I suspect it's the same for airline pilots—probably ninety-five percent of the time they are sitting in the cockpit looking at blue sky, the task of flying requiring only modest attention, but during takeoff and landing, or when significant status changes occur, focus is necessary. In air travel, however, a flight recorder is active. No such recordings are used in surgery, unless the surgeon requests to have a procedure videotaped. What *is* recorded (written) during every procedure is an anesthesiologist's detailed description of anesthetic events: when the anesthesia was administered, what type was used and at what dosage, what the patient's vital signs were at various intervals. Any pertinent discussions with the surgical team are also described, as are any concerns that were raised or any anesthetic interventions that occurred (such as placing monitoring devices or

CHAPTER 13 | *The Illness of Medicine*

making adjustments in ventilation equipment or intravenous or arterial access lines).

Similarly, the circulating nurse will record various matters during a procedure. These would include timed events (when the patient entered and left the operating room), any measures taken in regard to patient positioning and safety, and a pre- and postoperative inventory of all instruments, sponges, and needles brought into the operating room. The inventory is the primary means of ensuring that the postoperative instrument/sponge/needle count matches that of the preoperative count (in other words, that nothing got left in the patient). A surgical procedure is a dynamic event. As unanticipated developments occur, both innocuous and emergent, additional equipment may be required. If blood or blood products are given, a detailed record will be kept regarding the blood labels, the timing of administration, etc. A record is kept regarding all personnel in the surgical suite—who was present, and when they came and went. All of this notating is going on throughout the surgical case.

The surgery will generally proceed at the pace set by the surgeon in charge. Just as some individuals make decisions quickly while others require more deliberation, so do some surgeons assess problems quickly, deciding how to proceed and implement their plan, while others—slower in decision-making, sometimes painfully so—will debate with themselves and the assistants at the table what to do next. Speed is not to be confused with excellence. To be quick at something is not necessarily equivalent to doing something well. The highest-caliber surgeon understands that there are steps in a procedure that have little danger of complication and can be done more quickly. Other maneuvers are more delicate and have a significantly higher risk of causing damage (injury to blood vessels, nerves, organs). All doctors need to slow down the procedure to complete these particular segments carefully. There is certainly an "average" time necessary to complete a procedure. Unfortunately, I found that in today's corporate hospital structure, operating rooms most definitely included, the metrics used to measure "success" (e.g., time utilized to perform a procedure) are often wrong. Hospitals now measure down to the minute the time a surgeon takes to perform a particular operation. I completely disagree with the notion that a surgeon's skill or effectiveness can be measured by how fast he or she completes a procedure. Speed is *one* form of measurement, but I have seen very fast surgeons sometimes have less than desirable outcomes. However, the "hospital" (that is, the corporation) loves having that quick surgeon, because he or she allows the hospital to turn that operating room over to another case all the more quickly. After all, in the corporate world, time is money.

I remember once performing a robotically assisted laparoscopic radical prostatectomy. This is the laparoscopic removal of a cancerous prostate with the "assistance" of a precisely designed surgical robotic device. This sophisticated procedure requires advanced training and typically more operating-room time than an open prostatectomy, but it also offers several surgical advantages. I was having an issue in a particularly challenging case and was therefore slightly behind schedule (not to mention we had also started later than originally scheduled). During a delicate dissection segment

CHAPTER 13 | *The Illness of Medicine*

of the procedure, the head nurse of the operating room came in to see "how things were going." I informed her of our status, and of when I anticipated completing the case. This would mean that the operating room would now be behind schedule by about two hours. As I was peering into the robotic visual console to perform that difficult dissection, she felt it necessary to inform me that being behind in our schedule had consequences. She stated that the next patient would probably give us a "bad review" on their "patient survey" for being late. "Are you kidding me?" I responded. Was I actually supposed to go faster on this complicated case so that the survey might be more complimentary? Yes, because that survey is used by the hospital, and by hospital-review publications, as a mark of the hospital's "quality." Seriously.

The surgeon is trying to perform his best, but now the patient survey is dictating a quality "point scale" to be published in a hospital-review assessment. This will in turn be tabulated to help insurance companies determine which hospitals will or will not be "preferred." That status will in turn be used as a means of filling the hospital beds, which pays the bills and feeds the hospital hierarchy. But truly, the only really important outcome, in my assessment, was whether I cured the patient's cancer. I cared. The patient and his family cared. That is why he was there in the first place. But it appears that the hospital metrics that are judged by the insurance companies, by review consultants, and even by social-media evaluators have little, if anything, to do with procedure *outcomes*. Rather, they are based significantly on patient *perceptions* of treatment.

Michael J. Young, M.D.

I recall a surgeon who did more procedures than anyone else. I was convinced he would operate on a cadaver, if only he could figure out a way to bill for his services. To his shame, I never saw him turn down a case, regardless of any potential lack of expertise on his part. He would perform some pediatric procedures that, as in my field, just because I was boarded in pediatric urology, didn't mean I should go near certain complex situations. Many of those cases required the skills of a pediatric surgical specialist, one with additional training and an abundance of experience in these types of procedures. This surgeon was able to take on certain cases because, I suspect, the patient's parents didn't know the difference. He took on large oncologic (cancer) cases because he could, not because he should have. Unsurprisingly, his complication rate for some of these cases was higher than most. The residents who worked with him often found themselves alone in the OR, as he was letting them get the "feeling of being responsible." Not infrequently, he was reported to be eating "responsibly" in the doctor's lounge during these "teaching cases." A funny thing happened: He was offered a hospital's main managed-care contract. Apparently, quality of care was not the focal issue those hospital administrators sought. It was his speed of performing surgery, and his volume of cases, that they so highly valued.

Eventually, things did catch up, as they often do. His cancer cases were found to have higher than average positive margins, meaning cancerous cells were left behind after he'd ostensibly excised a tumor. Meetings were then established to help monitor surgical cases. The intent of these conferences was appropriate. But as a

CHAPTER 13 | *The Illness of Medicine*

means of curbing surgical judgment and behavior, the meetings themselves were less than productive. It is very difficult, if not impossible, to control when a "qualified" surgeon can operate. If patients come to a particular surgeon and agree to his plans and surgical recommendations, that is certainly their decision to make. But I do call on hospital administrators to act with more restraint in how they award their contracts.

* * * * * * * * * *

The final skin staples are applied. (Skin suturing has long been replaced by the use of staple guns and skin glues. The latter two are generally faster in application and leave quite acceptable results. Skin suturing is still an art/skill utilized by plastic surgeons and for specific procedures and circumstances.) Dressings are placed, and the patient is awakened by the anesthesiologist. It is truly remarkable how quickly modern anesthetic drugs can be reversed/metabolized. The patients often "wake up" now within minutes of the conclusion of surgery. They are taken into the recovery room, where a group of dedicated and often experienced nurses assume oversight of the patient. Vital signs are taken frequently, pain is managed, and a gradual return to mental normalcy occurs. The patients are then admitted for continued observation/management or, more frequently, they are discharged.

Michael J. Young, M.D.

When I started my urological training, in 1985, the average radical-prostatectomy patient was in the hospital seven days. When I completed my residency, in 1991, most patients could expect to be home around five to seven days following the procedure. By 1995, most patients were being sent home in four to five days. Five years after that, patients could expect to go home in three to four days. With the onset of robotically assisted prostate surgery in the early 2000s, many patients could expect to stay in the hospital just one night—and possibly an additional day, if necessary. This was a direct result not only of a much more minimally invasive procedure but also of much improved applications of fluid and pain management and an increased understanding of physiology and the healing process. Antibiotic usage, which previously was continued for weeks, was now being utilized for twenty-four hours. The overall speed of recovery had improved considerably. Consequently, patients were going home sooner—usually appropriately, but occasionally not.

Going home after surgery can be daunting. Patients will experience sensations they are not accustomed to. Prescribed medications will have potential side-effects. Things might be out of kilter. Bowel and bladder function may be affected by the anesthetics or analgesics (pain medication). One's eating and other routines and activities will take time to return to baseline. Physical assistance may be necessary. Add all of these issues to the psychological stresses that occur (fear of what happened, of an unwanted outcome, of job insecurity, of possible sexual dysfunction, etc.), and we have a considerable amount of anxiety.

CHAPTER 13 | *The Illness of Medicine*

Nevertheless, now you are to go home. The decision, really, has been predetermined for you: the insurance company says so. Yes, that company you have financed by dutifully paying your exorbitant premiums now dictates how much physical therapy you are entitled to, how long a visiting nurse can come to change your dressings and tend to your needs. What, you don't have a family member who can assist? Your wife *declines* to learn how to insert a catheter into your penis four times a day? She can't lift your 250 pounds onto the toilet? Per the insurance company, "What the hell is wrong with you?" This situation will now require innumerable phone calls, much paperwork, and ah yes, the all-important *referral*—that nonsensical piece of paper that states you have "approval" from some potentially clinically-inexperienced arbitrator (i.e., the medical director for the insurance company). His or her primary job, I believe, is first to say "no" and then see how far you or your advocates will push or complain. I have had many adversarial encounters with these "physicians" who work for and with the insurance company, whose salaries you underwrite with your premium payments. Good luck dealing with them!

So the surgery is now over, and recovery is proceeding. To say the process of having surgery is eventful is an understatement. I think being a patient in need of surgery can be one of the most difficult and worrisome situations. But despite all the potential complications, the vast majority of patients do get through the process and do get better, because the vast majority of surgeries are successful. If you need surgery, then get it. Trusting someone to operate on you can truly be a leap of faith. So learn the risks and do your due diligence to ensure, as best you can, not only that it is the right intervention for you but that you are being taken care of by the right person. There are many talented and devoted surgeons who perform and engage in these procedures every day. Make sure you understand the protocols and follow their directions. I honestly think you will be fine.

CHAPTER 14

Emergencies

The concept of what defines an emergency seems to differ among individuals. The perception of an emergency is also one that has evolved over the years, and changed with technological advances. Similarly, what causes a patient to go to an urgent care clinic, a hospital emergency room, or simply to his or her doctor's office varies greatly. Over years in practice, I witnessed these variables at play on a regular basis, and I reached a conclusion:

One factor that seems to have a significant role in the decision-making process of a patient with a perceived emergency is *time*.

I do not mean to imply that the patient understands the actual amount of time he has until his leg falls off from the injury he just sustained. Patients don't necessarily understand the severity of their problem. I mean the actual time it takes to get to be seen and how much of an inconvenience it is for the patient himself.

The ease with which physicians can be reached has also changed the perception of what constitutes an emergency. Years ago, if a patient had a medical problem—one that caused significant pain,

CHAPTER 14 | *The Illness of Medicine*

bleeding, or a change in mental status—he or she was brought into the hospital emergency room. With the advent of pagers, doctors became reachable no matter where they were. And with the advent of cell phones, patients could now reach out no matter where *they* were. It no longer mattered what time of day it was or whether any consideration had been given to the nature and severity (or harmlessness) of the actual "emergency." These days, if you have a question as to why your big toe is just a little bit swollen, well, time to pull out the phone and satisfy your need to know, *now*. Yes, people can be that demanding. On many occasions, they are insensitive to the invasion of the doctor's life. They may, and will, be calling you at midnight or on Sunday morning. They are your patient, and they feel entitled to call. It's just so easy to reach the doctor, who now has to drop what he's doing to answer your call. Most calls are not emergencies at all.

Just the other day, I was having dinner with an old friend who is a dermatologist. It was a Friday evening, after a long day, and week, for him. During the meal, he was interrupted with a page. Abruptly, he stopped what he was doing and tended to the call. The patient was a young woman who thought she noted a slight change in a freckle on her arm. During the conversation, she apparently told him she didn't know how long ago she noted the change. "Maybe a week or so?" I overheard him repeat to her. She was concerned it could be melanoma. Really. That couldn't have waited until the next business day? The patients panic. In a short-fused, demanding, entitled society, our technology has enabled this behavior. A total lack of consideration for anything or anyone other than oneself

Michael J. Young, M.D.

has emerged—a lack of consideration and a lack of judgment that I doubt will ever be acknowledged.

Many "emergency" calls are inevitably at night. Not that the actual problem occurred at night, but night is when patients have the *time* to call. They have been at work all day, and it isn't until the evening/night hours that they have the ability to make the call. I can appreciate this. What I can't appreciate is the fact that patients will have had the problem for days or possibly weeks before deciding to call *at night*. If the doctor dares suggest a visit to the emergency room (ER), the patients turn from fearful to angry. Why, they feel, should they have to wait in an ER? (Why, they never seem to ask themselves, did they wait for days or weeks only to call the doctor after hours?) No, they don't have time to go to the ER at that "time" (i.e., after hours). ERs are typically a mess at night. Why? Because everyone has done the same thing—they've waited until after work, when it's more convenient to address the problem that has been nagging them for who knows how long. From what most of my patients shared with me, the typical time spent in an ER is about four hours, for the most routine of problems.

In an attempt to save time, a fair number of patients will skip the hospital ER and go to their local urgent care clinic instead. Such clinics are conveniently located in a variety of both large and small strip malls. These centers promise quick in-and-out care, and typically, that's what the patients receive. In my experience, unless it's a relatively simple, straight-forward condition, rarely is the problem fully addressed by these centers. Rather, treatment most often consists of a pain medication, an antibiotic (needed or not),

CHAPTER 14 | *The Illness of Medicine*

and a recommendation that patients see their doctor ASAP. Urgent care clinics have very limited imaging capability. They might be able to perform a plain x-ray or ultrasound examination, and only some are able to perform a computed tomography (CT) scan, which urologists, for instance, often rely on to obtain precise information regarding most urological conditions (bleeding from the urinary tract, the presence and location of possible kidney stones, etc.). If the physician on duty at one of these centers were reasonably trained, he or she could place an indwelling Foley catheter for patients experiencing urinary retention (inability to urinate). A Foley catheter is a type of tube that is placed through the urethra into the bladder to facilitate the emptying of the bladder. It can also be used to irrigate, or flush, the bladder if necessary. But again, if the patient has a moderately complex urological history, or previous history of urological surgery, the case may be beyond the capabilities of an urgent care clinic. Personally, I would not go to one of these centers unless I had something of a well-known issue (for instance, cold symptoms, or a simple laceration or a minor injury). Anything potentially complex may receive little more than a superficial evaluation—not necessarily because of any ineptness but simply as a consequence of the often limited clinical resources at these centers. I have seen significant problems improperly evaluated and potentially life-threatening conditions not recognized at these in-and-out clinics. I'm sure they fill a void in the overall health care equation, but perhaps more so in specialties other than urology. My experience with them was one of inconsistent care and hit-or-miss diagnoses.

Michael J. Young, M.D.

The hospital emergency room, typically far superior in both its regulation and its available resources, is a better place to go for an emergency urological evaluation. It will not be quick, or cheap, but most often, the problem will be resolved or stabilized. From the standpoint of a urological surgeon, dealing with the ER can at times be challenging. Part of the problem is that ER physicians are trained to handle a variety of problems—from diaper rash to an acute heart attack or stroke. Consequently, their level of understanding of the details of each specialty will be limited. However, although they may not be able to place a Foley catheter any better than the staff at the urgent care center, they do have access to specialists. Every hospital ER has a roster of specialists on call, for problems the hospital staff members can't resolve or handle themselves. One of my complaints toward the end of my years practicing was that I saw an increased frequency of these calls, only because the ER attending hadn't even tried to resolve the problem. Too many ER physicians just pick up the phone and call someone for help, when in fact they should at least try to resolve the problem first, and call only in the event of failure.

Male patients typically wait until the last minute before calling the doctor. Perhaps this is related to the fact that men don't regularly see their physician, whereas women have annual gynecological exams. Once the male patient is finally dragged into the office by his companion, who has grown tired of his complaining, he behaves as if this is a first-time experience. Maybe it is. If I walked into an exam room to see a female patient, I could let her know what to do (undress, put on a gown) and then return with one of

CHAPTER 14 | *The Illness of Medicine*

my female medical assistants confident that the patient would be ready for examination. Were the patient male, I could offer the same instructions and then return five minutes later to find that *maybe* his belt would be undone. Okay, let's try this again. Five minutes later maybe the shirt would be unbuttoned. Whatever.

A particular oddity I encountered when taking telephone calls regarding male-patient emergencies: The caller was almost always *the wife*.

This was the strangest thing. The patient's wife would call, and I could hear the patient telling his wife what to say: Tell the doctor it hurts here, or that it hurts when I do this or that. To obtain more information, I would then ask the wife some questions, and she would in turn ask her husband for the answers. He would respond, and she would convey the answers back to me. This continued, typically, until I ran out of patience and asked to speak directly to the patient. Then he, the patient, would take over the call as if she, the wife, had simply been incapable of properly communicating his condition. This phenomenon happened year after year, call after call.

The diligent wife would do her best to describe her husband's problem to the doctor, and would later make his appointments, ensuring that he followed up. On the other hand, if the wife were the patient with a problem, she typically called for herself.

One of the more frustrating problems with an emergency call was that the patient wouldn't respond as instructed. This was not my problem, except that it inevitably meant the patient would show up later with a worsened condition. The patient who would call on a Monday (night) for a problem and then wouldn't actually show until Thursday afternoon was not uncommon. This became a significant inconvenience for me as I now had to squeeze this patient in somewhere in my already packed schedule. Because of the patient's failure to come in earlier for evaluation, as previously recommended, his problem had been allowed to deteriorate further, and other appointments now had to be rescheduled, canceled, or delayed to accommodate this particular individual's more urgent needs. It's one thing if a true emergency comes in. It's another thing entirely if, based upon the patient's own selfishness or disregard for instruction, he lumbers into the ER or the office at the last minute, a time that happens to be convenient for him, and forces everyone else (patients and staff alike) to adjust. This certainly does not endear the patient to the doctor. More important, it wears the doctor out. He simply reaches a point where, because of this and everything else going on in the medical profession, he decides to stop practicing medicine.

CHAPTER 15

Medical Marketing

When I was growing up the medical world appeared to be a sacred place. On television, the shows about hospitals, doctors, and medical frontiers were filled with episodes of drama, heroism, and intense decision-making. The doctors would be seen deliberating over or arguing about what the absolute best treatment for the patient would be. The tension often reached such a pitch that I was exhausted at the conclusion of a show. Life and death hung in the balance in scenes from emergency rooms. No simple splinters were being removed in these ERs; only absolute trauma and blood-transfusion-type events were portrayed. Even the residents on television would jump into the most complex circumstances to save a life. Nurses outfitted in caps and white uniforms answered doctors' and patients' questions with undivided attention and thorough knowledge. Near-death experiences were often featured in scenes from the operating room. This was serious stuff! Medicine was serious. The people were serious.

Fast-forward to today: We are no longer watching television shows depicting the extraordinary bravery and compassion of medical

CHAPTER 15 | *The Illness of Medicine*

professionals. Today's medical shows appear less focused on clinical issues and more closely resemble an alternative type of soap opera. In these dramas, medicine is just a narrative device around which to weave somewhat overwrought, complex, interpersonal conundrums of the sort I never encountered in my years in medicine. The stories and events are often just so unbelievable. But people love them. *Grey's Anatomy* is in its fourteenth season and counting; *ER* ran for fifteen years (from the mid-1990s to 2009); *House* had an eight-year run, ending less than five years ago. *Chicago Med, Code Black,* and others are currently running. But the visceral excitement I remember in medical shows has been replaced with so much fluff. These contemporary works are often more like melodramas than medical dramas. As we have drifted away from the heroism and greater realism of older medical shows on television, we have also seen television become a sales and marketing outlet for the health care industry. Exaggerated medical dramas of more recent vintage have, however unintentionally, helped prepare us for the next natural sequence of medicine on TV: health care and pharmaceutical advertising.

This new era of medical marketing can be very dangerous. You've seen the ads and heard the promises. I've seen the results. Medicine and medical treatment can't and should not be marketed like a new luxury item. Health care in America accounts for approximately one-sixth of the gross domestic product, and the ad campaigns of those competing within the industry contribute their share to that impressive total. The thing hospitals and pharmaceutical companies typically don't advertise is the cost of their new therapies. And cost is ultimately the greatest barrier to treatment.

Michael J. Young, M.D.

One of the hospitals in Illinois promoted its services on a billboard with the slogan, "Emergencies Happen." How cute. How clever. How insensitive.

Yes, emergencies do happen. But if you are the patient who has just suffered a stroke, had a heart attack, or fallen from a ladder and fractured your spine, somehow the advertising company paid to come up with such a ridiculous slogan doesn't seem so clever. Real people enduring genuinely catastrophic events are looking for a place that provides quality help, not cheap sloganeering. More bothersome to me was that the ER being advertised just was not stellar, in my opinion. My suspicion is that its staff would have had difficulty diagnosing hiccups if you walked in the door actually hiccupping. "No, wait, let's first get a CT scan. Then we'll call your primary M.D. to see if this has happened before. It could be indicative of something else." Or, you know, it might be hiccups. None of that old TV glamor here.

What's really annoying are the numerous advertisements that hospitals and medical centers strategically place among TV entertainment. It has become a war of nonsensical comparisons, of polling percentages displaying which hospital among those that advertise is ranked highest for this or that procedure, or according to this or that metric. Each hospital portrays itself as the epicenter of advanced medical research. Considering that probably ninety-five percent of medical problems don't require the resources of such advanced facilities, it seems frivolous to spend enormous amounts of money advertising to the person at home, who is probably drinking a beer and watching a baseball game when the ad appears. But let's consider how much it did cost to write, direct, produce, and then buy air time for the typical

CHAPTER 15 | *The Illness of Medicine*

ad, which shows (for instance) "scientific" test tubes containing cool blue liquid spinning around in a centrifuge under the watchful eye of an actress in a white lab coat and protective goggles. That blue liquid is clearly some magical potion being created by the geniuses at that research facility. If they can do that, surely that is the place where I want to have my liposuction performed. Oddly, I have never seen or heard any of these advertisements address the cost of their wondrous treatment.

Indeed, what is most insane about all of this medical-center advertising is that there is a significant impediment to most people's being treated at such places. Just because a hospital portrays itself as the pinnacle of medical knowledge and the core of scientific research does not mean that the gatekeepers of American health care—the insurance companies—will allow most patients to seek treatment there. A hospital or medical center may advance itself on television or radio until every last million is spent, but if a person can't get a referral to go there, well, I guess he or she won't be visiting the home of the special blue liquid in test tubes anytime soon. Again, which specialist, hospital, or treatment center you may go to is dependent upon your PPO or HMO plan. Personally, I am finding that understanding which group you are enrolled in is as confusing as figuring out which boarding group you're in at the airline gate: are you platinum, gold, emerald, preferred, executive, priority, or preferred executive, or are you like the rest of us who simply ride coach and get tossed a bag of peanuts? It is not only difficult to understand, but nearly impossible to negotiate. I had patients who were among the few percent who had unique medical problems, patients who truly needed treatment at an advanced center or with a particular specialist. But because that center or specialist was not in this or that patient's insurance plan, and because the medical director for the insurance company appeared primarily concerned with protecting his bonus by not allowing "outside" referrals, these patients were committed to their local treatment centers.

My disdain for pharmaceutical advertising is even more difficult to contain. How many pills do pharmaceutical companies have to sell in order to cover the hundreds of millions, if not billions, of dollars they spend in advertising? I can't watch the news or a golf match on television without the constant bombardment of these commercials, each one trying to be more amazing than the last. These commercials generally come in two varieties: the serious and the not-so-serious. The serious ads show computer-generated images of body parts and how the new drug reduces inflammation, withers infection, or shrinks a tumor. The voice actor narrating the ad will employ a rich baritone as he describes the miracle of events. The language will be infused with medical jargon and accompanied by a significant use of graphs and numbers to amaze and astound the observer, who is really more interested in watching professional wrestling late at night. Few viewers, if any, actually understand the medical lingo, but it sure sounds authoritative. Even with all my training, I don't understand much of the medical doubletalk. The deep baritone voice reviews the side effects of a new cancer drug: "You may experience capillary leak syndrome," like this symptom or condition is common knowledge.

On the other end of the advertising spectrum one finds attempts at humor, but watching an actress run around dressed up as a colon, a bladder, or a nostril does not inspire me to call my physician for a new prescription. These ads are not only silly but also, frankly, insulting.

CHAPTER 15 | *The Illness of Medicine*

After the usual ridiculous short story of disease is played out, the bulk of a typical ad is spent on legal disclaimers spoken in hushed tones very quickly. Recently I was able to watch several of these ads during a single television program. A scenario they all had in common was one I never witnessed in nearly three decades of practice: a physician actually sitting with a patient as—together—they reviewed the medical indications/treatment on an iPad or other computer device. Who has the time for that? Given that the doctor probably has only two and a half minutes to discuss the problem and only two and a half minutes to examine the patient, and must spend nearly ten minutes typing up the evaluation in the medical record, does the doctor really sit down with the patient to watch the product video? Then the ads showed the physician personally escorting the patient into the corridor of the office building. In what world do these advertising producers live? And how come these patients are seen romping in a park, or dancing, because their psoriasis is better? Ridiculous.

However, the erectile-dysfunction ads take the prize. The gorgeous model wearing the blue men's shirt, lying on the blue sheets, and advertising the little blue pill—it's all as subtle as a caveman's club. As for another drug company's marketing ploy, despite my training, education, and life experiences, I simply cannot figure out why two people sitting in adjacent white porcelain bathtubs are a symbol of sexual activity.

And after being subjected to all this marketing crap, even if you did decide that you couldn't live without the new drug, well, guess what? That drug you now desire and really know nothing about except perhaps that it can induce flatulence if not taken properly (that's what they said on TV) cannot be prescribed to you per your insurance prescription plan unless it is on the pharmaceutical formulary determined by your insurance. And should you decide to go off formulary, meaning you will get the drug with a prescription from your doctor and not go through your insurance plan, well, hold on tight. A treatment's worth of that new miracle elixir will require a loan from the bank. Indigestion will be the least of its side effects, as poverty might now set in. These new drugs are exorbitantly expensive, as are—not incidentally—the ads that promote their use. And so the circle continues. The patient, again, serves as a conduit for the flow of money within the system.

Of course, given the competitive nature of the "business" of medicine, doctors themselves are advertising too. Does anyone really pay attention to the printed ad found in an airline's inflight magazine showing the "best doctors in America"? Are these really the best, or perhaps just the ones who paid for the opportunity to be promoted in their best suit and matching pocket kerchief? I was once included in a local magazine listing the "best physicians." A funny thing happened the following year. I was called by the publisher of the magazine to ask if I wanted to be in it again. I thought inclusion was based on an honor system, not a payment plan.

A physician I knew of demonstrated blatant disregard for the decorum once required when addressing a certain medical issue. During the late 1990s he took out a billboard along one of the major highways near Chicago with only one word on it, in large, block letters: "IMPOTENT?" This was followed by his office number. The sign was in bright yellow, and the lettering was in black. You simply

CHAPTER 15 | *The Illness of Medicine*

could not miss it unless you were driving in the opposite direction. It was offensive and obnoxious. It seemed to me that some fundamental law of nature had been broken when this sign went up. It was the first time I saw a doctor taking out not just this kind of an advertisement, but one of colossal proportions.

What subsequently disturbed me even more was the consequence of this ad. I recall being called to the emergency room one evening to see a middle-aged Cambodian man writhing in pain. His wife, twenty years his junior, was there with him. He'd seen the "IMPOTENT?" billboard and, despite having no sexual dysfunction, had made an appointment to see the doctor in question. The physician had subsequently convinced the man that although he was not suffering any erectile dysfunction at the time, he would need help eventually given the age discrepancy with his younger wife. The patient told me that the doctor's office helped him set up a payment plan, and a penile prosthesis was implanted.

A penile prosthesis is essentially a semirigid or inflatable silicone device that is implanted inside of the penis. It adds rigidity to the penis for sexual activity. These are ingenious mechanical devices that work exceptionally well, and for the appropriate patients—those who truly do have erectile dysfunction that cannot be treated by less invasive methods—they are a godsend. However, one of the more serious risks of any surgical implantation is postoperative infection. And that is just what the Cambodian patient experienced: a serious infection that mandated immediate removal of the device on the night I was called. Unfortunately, once such a serious infection occurs, significant scar tissue can develop. The patient, who'd never had erectile dysfunction, now had a permanent case of it from the postoperative complication of a procedure that never should have been performed in the first place. He'd been perfectly fine when he first saw that billboard, now, as a consequence of calling the number on it, he truly was "IMPOTENT." A well-placed advertisement had attracted a vulnerable patient and directed him to a self-promoting physician.

Is this any less objectionable than the lawyer who advertises that he should be consulted if someone experiences a slip and fall—or a bad medical outcome? I suspect they are both trying to take advantage of needy, frightened, or gullible clients. When presented properly, good marketing can probably induce even the most careful and conservative people to undertake things that are completely outrageous.

We all have weak moments, and are at risk—under the right circumstances—of making a wrong decision. Although I may disagree with many of the messages the advertisers are conveying, my main concern is that the target of medical marketing—the patient—is usually at a vulnerable moment in his or her life, dealing with a medical issue. The advertisers are taking full advantage of that moment. Proper health care is a precious commodity, yet a mistake in its management can often have lifelong repercussions. If hospitals and pharmaceutical companies are to be allowed to advertise, they need to be genuinely responsible about informing patients of *appropriate* management. They shouldn't be allowed to make a perfunctory show of responsibility simply as a way of masking their real intent, which is to promote a product for sale.

CHAPTER 16

Mistakes

We all make mistakes. By definition, they are not intentional, yet despite all efforts to avoid them, they will inevitably occur. Booking the wrong flight, applying the wrong paint, backing into the garage door, are all mistakes, and we beat ourselves up about making them. Unfortunately, in a hospital/medical environment, the consequences of a mistake can be life-altering or even fatal. During my years in practice, I learned that the great majority of errors could easily have been avoided. It doesn't take a new computer program or a great deal of time or a great number of steps to be preventative in one's approach. It really just takes common sense. I'm not sure that a lack of common sense is anything new, but what *is* new, I feel, is the amount of distraction, multitasking, and overextending that occurs in the modern workplace and that is a significant contributor to errors. A hospital environment, given its complexity of services and the frequent urgency with which they're provided, can lend itself to error. But again, reviewing error after error, the common theme is that nobody really took the time to simply think through what he or she was doing just prior to the event occurring.

CHAPTER 16 | *The Illness of Medicine*

One example of a failure to think, an example that simply boggles the mind, involves two patients who underwent prostate biopsies. A standard prostate biopsy is a procedure (usually performed to assess if cancer is present) in which a hollow needle is placed through the rectum and into the prostate gland in order to obtain a sampling of the tissue, which is then evaluated under a microscope by a pathologist. Generally, multiple "cores" are taken, placed into specimen cups, and sent to the pathology department. The procedure takes roughly fifteen minutes and can be performed under local anesthesia.

I suspect my practice was similar to other busy medical practices. I had patients with unique names and many patients with common names. Interestingly, I had many patients with the same first and last names. Sometimes, only by referring to a middle initial or date of birth could I distinguish the records of patients who had the same names. On occasion, I had two patients with the same name come into the office on the same day for regular follow-up appointments. The appointments had been scheduled at different times, possibly months apart, and only by mere chance had both patients appeared in my office on the same day. That happens.

Here's what shouldn't happen. A surgeon's office should never schedule two patients with the same first and last names to undergo the same procedure on the same day at the same hospital. That is just asking for trouble. And the idiocy of such scheduling did indeed result in trouble. A urologist in another state had two patients with exactly the same name scheduled for prostate biopsies on the same day. The biopsies themselves were uneventful. That is, no complications occurred. When the pathology reports came in,

Michael J. Young, M.D.

one patient was diagnosed with prostate cancer and the other was not. Consequently, the patient with prostate cancer was counseled on treatment options and apparently elected to have a radical prostatectomy. This is a major surgical procedure with the potential for serious complications. At the very least, the quality of one's future erections will most likely be affected, and incontinence may occur. The patient underwent his prostatectomy, and—interestingly—on his final pathology report, no cancer was identified. He'd been "cured," even before the prostatectomy.

The other lucky chap who did not have cancer on his pathology report went about his way and never had any treatment. But, of course, he was the one who actually had the cancer. The biopsy samples had been mixed up.

Yes, there were errors made up and down the line. The samples should never have been mixed up in the first place. Proper handling of the specimens should have involved not just a name but also another identifier, such as a birth date or medical record number. But why had the doctor's office scheduled the same procedure to be done at the same hospital, on patients with the same name, on the same day? Were the doctor's staffers at fault? Well, they weren't the ones who actually mixed up the samples. But couldn't someone in the office have recognized the potential for a problem and simply put one of the biopsies on a different day? As we hear so often, common sense isn't so common.

While on the subject of prostatectomy, let's discuss in a bit more detail what is actually being performed during this procedure. The prostate gland is a walnut-sized gland that lives between the urinary bladder

CHAPTER 16 | *The Illness of Medicine*

and the urethra (the tube through which urine flows out of the penis). After removal of the prostate, the reconstruction requires that the urethra be attached to the bladder. A catheter is placed into the urethra and through to the bladder, to essentially stabilize the anastomosis (the attachment) during the healing process. The catheter is held in place by a small inflatable "balloon" that is part of the tubing at its tip inside the bladder. This prevents the tube from being dislodged. The balloon can be inflated or deflated through a small port at the external end of the catheter. The catheter will be left in place for approximately one to two weeks to allow the anastomosis to heal, depending upon how the procedure was performed.

Prior to robotic surgery, and still a method preferred today by some surgeons, the prostate gland was removed in an "open" fashion, meaning through an incision. Some fifteen years ago, I performed an open radical prostatectomy on a very kind and gentle man in his mid-sixties. He was the type of patient who would never complain. He always followed instructions and always followed up. He was a delight to treat, and his surgery had gone very well. Everyone was pleased. The day after his prostate surgery, I walked into his room on morning rounds expecting to see my patient in the early stage of a fine recovery. Instead, what I found was that his catheter had been removed earlier. I went ballistic. I found out that a new nursing student had removed the catheter. But how could that have come about? How could someone, a new student no less, have thought it wise to take out a component that plays such an integral role in the recovery from this procedure? Who gave this student the order to do this? Who but I even had the authority to give such an order? The young nursing student had been told to remove the Foley catheter on Mr. Johnson (not his actual name), but as it happens, there were two Mr. Johnsons—in *adjacent* rooms. She had gotten the room numbers mixed up. I remember my thoughts of retaliation as I wheeled my patient to the x-ray department so that we could try to reinsert the necessary catheter under fluoroscopy (live x-ray). I was so upset with the current state of affairs for my patient. But under x-ray, we were indeed able to replace the tube without incident, and my patient just took it all in stride, like he did everything else. He was fine. I was not. But after calming down, I realized that the student was just following orders: Take the catheter out of Mr. Johnson. The system, again, had failed. A mistake occurred because of human error, a breakdown in proper patient identification similar to the error in the prostate biopsies. Fortunately, in the catheter event, the mistake was quickly identified and rectified. But to eliminate similar events in the future would require a restructuring of how patient-identification procedures are performed.

In surgery, it can be quite confusing when multiple procedures of the same type are being performed all day on the same organ. For instance, an ophthalmologist may perform a dozen cataract procedures in a single day. Going from the right eye on one patient to the left and then the right again on subsequent patients lends itself to error. In addition, if a patient is "draped," meaning covered except for the incision site, a surgeon walking into an operating room may make an incision and inadvertently remove, say, the good kidney instead of the cancerous one. In recognition of the possibility of such errors, methods have been implemented and evolved over time to minimize the likelihood of mistakes. For instance, repeated verification of operation site and side has become mandatory in operating rooms.

CHAPTER 16 | *The Illness of Medicine*

Site markings (in which the surgeon draws with a pen or marker on the actual limb, or side, that the upcoming surgery will be performed) are also required. A "time-out" is called prior to any procedure so that all operating-room personnel can stop and take a moment to agree that they have the required equipment and the right patient, and that the right procedure is about to be performed on the correct side. This type of "check listing" protocol is performed in many industries—for instance, air travel. Pilots go through a list of mandatory preflight steps to ensure thorough operational safety. Why it took the medical profession so long to adopt such protocols is unclear.

One of the more complex problems in modern medicine is the explosion of new drugs. As a prescribing physician, simply trying to keep up with this ever changing medicinal formulary is a challenge. Consequently, knowing all of the indications, side effects, and drug interactions is difficult, if not impossible. The drug names alone, born of marketing fancy, are bewildering. Keeping everything straight can be confusing. Often, patients are on multiple drugs, adding to the confusion: Flonase to help you breathe, Flomax to help you urinate, and so on. If you add in the generics (the cost-saving alternatives to exorbitantly priced brand-name medications), patients might come into the office or hospital with a laundry list of medications that can be difficult to decipher.

I was once consulted on a patient for urinary retention—he couldn't urinate. The patient was on multiple medications, for Parkinson's, for depression, and two additional drugs to minimize urinary frequency. Was it any wonder he couldn't pee? His primary physician admitted him to the hospital. What the patient really needed was to have someone carefully go over his list of drugs and the doctor suggest that instead of adding new drugs he might consider weaning the patient off of some of the ones he is already taking. Had the prescribing physician not taken the appropriate time to simply review the patient's medication list? Perhaps it is just easier to write a prescription (and now upgrade one's billing) than to eliminate one of the dozen daily drugs a patient may be taking. It takes time to review a chart. When the average primary physician seems to have about fifteen minutes per patient (must maintain the volume to keep the salary and bonus), mistakes will happen.

A word about EMRs (electronic medical records). As with nearly every form of human interactivity today, digitalization is particularly common within the health profession. As I drive to work, and nearly hit pedestrians walking across the street fixated on their smart phones and not on what is happening around them, it is obvious that our lives are not always improved by these wondrous digital tools. Rather, in many ways, we are controlled by them. The digitalization of our lives must of course be accepted as the new norm. And in the medical profession, the advantages of these technological resources are obvious. No longer do medical offices need to have precious (and often very costly) space set aside to store voluminous charts and records—records that undoubtedly have some pages that are illegible, faded, or lost. With electronic records, everyone can now read what is entered. Nothing is lost. Unfortunately, if the wrong information is inadvertently added, correcting the error may not be as easy. The mistake will keep recurring each and every time that medical record is transferred, replicated, or even just printed. But it's not just the actual

CHAPTER 16 | The Illness of Medicine

record that might be in error and in need of correction. Also in need of correction is the process through which *corrections themselves* must be made, a process that can be difficult if not impossible to navigate. Layers of information (and personnel) must be negotiated in order to facilitate a simple change.

As an example, I had a patient with bladder cancer I must have treated nearly twenty years prior. Bladder tumors basically come in two varieties: those that are considered relatively benign and that have a low probability of progression and invasion into the deeper layers of the bladder, and those that when found are already into the deep muscle of the bladder and are considered aggressive. The latter have a significant potential to metastasize, or invade other locations. The treatment and management of these two types of tumors are vastly different. The more benign, superficial tumors are scraped out and are generally subject to frequent cystoscopic evaluations (involving a light and camera that are placed into the bladder to observe the inside of the bladder). On some occasions, drugs are placed into the bladder to help control the tumor. The tumors that have grown into the bladder muscle typically result in the bladder itself having to be removed—a major surgical procedure.

Years ago, medical conditions were assigned an identification number, a code, that was part of a larger classification system meant to facilitate billing, to streamline insurance processes, and to more efficiently record/identify a medical condition. The system had (obvious) inaccuracies and has undergone extensive revision since its implementation. We are now at a point where the coding of medical conditions is much more detailed, including not only the disease itself but also such specifics as its extent, size, and/or location. Twenty years ago, I would simply insert into the billing/labeling record the code indicating that my patient had a "bladder tumor."

Years after the event, the patient who'd had the bladder tumor called. She was doing well—no medical problems—but she wanted her medical records to more clearly state that her bladder tumor had been of the superficial variety and not the more aggressive variety. Her previous diagnostic coding had simply been one of "bladder cancer." I hadn't heard from her in years, so the call was a bit surprising, but perhaps she was applying for new health insurance. I set out to do as she asked, feeling that her request was certainly appropriate: to provide a more updated and accurate diagnostic code for her previous condition. Interestingly, I couldn't do it. The EMR would not let me swap out the old code for the new. Oh, I could modify her record so that the newer coding description was in there, too, but I could not eliminate the less accurate, older code. It made me think about the consequences if I had put in the wrong diagnosis the first time. When it comes to EMRs, once it's in there, it's in there. Accurate or not, it stays there, to be replicated and reproduced by anyone who touches the record.

Another issue of concern regarding the use of electronic medical records is the fact that billing is tied into documentation. This means that a physician can bill only for documented treatment. If I perform a procedure on a patient and submit a bill to insurance (essentially, submit a list of coded numbers representing the actual interventions performed), the insurance company may ask for the operative

CHAPTER 16 | *The Illness of Medicine*

report, which is a dictated description of events that occurred during the procedure, to verify that the submission of the billing codes is justified. In the view of the insurance company (and speaking medico-legally), if it isn't documented, it didn't happen—even though I may have performed something that I simply failed to dictate into the operative report.

Just as bothersome is that the scrupulously maintained EMR is not always truthful, or necessarily accurate. In other words, the EMR programs are designed to document. To facilitate and streamline documentation, these programs typically have bulk parameters that the physician simply has to click on in order to verify that something was done. Say a patient comes into the office for an exam. The provider will talk to the patient, perform a perfunctory exam, and then document what was done. He may click on a button indicating that the entire exam is "normal." In just a fraction of a second, with a single click, the head exam, abdominal exam, chest exam, and extremity exam are recorded evermore as having been "normal" on this day in history. Did he really examine those areas in detail, as the click was meant to indicate? Unlikely. However, now that all those body parts have ostensibly been checked, he can bill for their examination. The detailed exam wasn't really performed, but documenting it in the EMR suffices to *prove* that it was.

So, underdocumentation (a failure to dictate all aspects of a procedure) results in lack of appropriate payment, and overdocumentation ensures payment for services that are potentially not actually performed. The former is a mistake. The latter, depending on intent, can border on fraud and regardless of intent will result in additional billing and likely additional and inappropriate payment. Most important, the overdocumentation results in a potentially inaccurate description of that patient's condition. Unfortunately, I have witnessed this overdocumentation in the EMR all too often, not only on physicians' office records but throughout hospital EMR systems as well. There is simply no possible way—as recorded in many a patient's EMR, in sections pertaining to admission history and physical exam—that every system (respiratory, circulatory, musculoskeletal, etc.) was examined to the degree each is documented to have been. I saw physicians in the hospital rounding in and out of patient rooms in literally minutes, yet for the record ten or twelve medical evaluations were noted as having been performed. It is simply not possible. Not only is this a misrepresentation in billing, involving charging for services not provided, but more important, such inaccurate recording of what really was examined or done during an evaluation can have adverse medical consequences. It can allow abnormalities to go undetected longer than they should—because others might subsequently skip examining systems coded as "normal," on the assumption that these systems have truly, recently been examined and found healthy.

For instance, if nobody actually did a twelve-point exam (meaning look at twelve health systems on the patient), but this is documented as having been done, no further exams of these areas are likely to be performed. Why repeat examining something that is already noted in the record as being "normal"? The time-tested medical-record notation "WNL," meaning "within normal limits," would now more accurately imply "we never looked." But in the current EMR programs, things marked "normal" are truly thought to have been

CHAPTER 16 | *The Illness of Medicine*

examined. I saw countless EMRs describing a "normal" prostate. Yet if I asked the patient about his exam, it would transpire that nobody had performed a rectal exam, which is the only palpable means of determining if the prostate is truly normal. But it was documented as so. If a malignancy were present, nobody would know, and the patient record would be completely inaccurate.

Certainly, one explanation for this problem, and it's not an excuse, would be that physicians are now required to see so many patients in such limited time that these shortcuts are inevitable. If such shortcuts are nothing but a sly means of padding a bill for reimbursement, then they are inexcusable and frankly dangerous, since they could be putting the patient in harm's way. But even if such notations are a kind of mistake, or are indicative of nothing more than sloppy practice patterns, the potential consequences are the same. Regardless of intent or lack of intent, we need better "intelligence" in managing how we provide health care and how we document that care.

Most important, if we are going to minimize mistakes in medicine, we need to take a long look at what we are doing and why we are doing it. We need integrity. We need to slow down. We also need to take the drive for financial consideration out of the equation for health care.

CHAPTER 17

Cancer

Conveying a cancer diagnosis to a patient was one of the most challenging issues I confronted in clinical practice. How patients reacted to the diagnosis and to the management of their problem varied. The situation required careful, deliberate consideration on the doctor's part. I have read countless articles and books, and attended numerous lectures and symposia, on cancer-discussion management. Yet despite all that preparation and study, what it really came down to was having an honest rapport with the patient. Through all the possible changes in the disease progression and all the corresponding changes in the patient's emotional state, a sustainable, dependable relationship is mandatory. The patients will be elated with a positive response to treatment, and in deep despair at news of failure. Both conditions must be addressed with a level-headed patience. Above all, one must be a good listener.

In my urological practice, cancer diagnoses occurred in one of two basic scenarios. In the first scenario, patients who were otherwise feeling great were found to have a laboratory or imaging abnormality consistent with cancer. In the other scenario, patients

CHAPTER 17 | *The Illness of Medicine*

came in because they were already feeling ill, but for reasons unknown. Understanding how these two different groups of patients would likely adjust to their findings and work through the various stages of treatment required not only a thorough knowledge of the natural history of the disease itself but also of human behavior. I don't believe this type of empathy can be taught. Think of the difference between those who merely know how to use a camera to take pictures and those who, using the very same equipment, possess the ability to compose photographs that convey emotion and understanding. Most physicians learn the mechanics of cancer treatment—how to follow a protocol of therapy. But few know how to actually *listen* to the patient with the disease, the better to learn the patient's perspective and tailor the treatment to the patient's level of understanding and emotional tolerance. Treating the patient *with* the disease—rather than treating the disease that happens to be in the patient—is critical.

I found that medical oncologists, specialists in the medical management of cancer, and radiation oncologists, those who treat cancer with radiation therapy, were generally better in discussing with patients their status and treatment regimens than were most surgeons who treated cancer. Perhaps it was a consequence of their training. Perhaps it was simply that certain personality types migrate into each of those specialties. Obviously, there were exceptions. I also knew some truly stupendous urologic oncologic surgeons who understood how to discuss their clinical findings clearly and empathetically with a patient. They just seemed to be a rare breed.

I always made it my practice to discuss a patient's cancer diagnosis initially with the patient alone, and then encourage the inclusion of the patient's family or significant other in the discussion. Cancer often requires months, if not years, of treatment and management for potential recovery. The disease affects everyone close to that patient. And for that reason, I felt that everyone who would be immediately involved in care should be kept informed on the process of treatment. Ultimately, however, whether or not to include others in such discussions was something only the patient had the right to decide.

I am not a psychiatrist, but I did observe the mental and emotional processes that patients would undergo with their cancer diagnoses. These involved the classic reactions to grief: denial, anger, bargaining, depression, and acceptance.

The intensity of a patient's reactions could also be related to how the diagnosis came about. The patient coming in, say, for a discussion about an abnormal blood test who is otherwise going about daily activities has a much harder time accepting his diagnosis. He will deny the reality of it, sometimes to the point of failing even to return for continued discussion or management. This does not appear to be a consequence of misunderstanding. It is simply how some choose to deal—or, rather, not deal—with an unwelcome development.

Interestingly, I also noticed that the acceptance of a cancer diagnosis was frequently related to a patient's socioeconomic status. Wealthier patients seemed to be able to dismiss the news as one of those errors that are simply beyond one's control. Perhaps it was the result of a mistaken diagnosis (something that was not uncommonly insinuated). Many would immediately request copies of their records as they planned their soliciting of second opinions—

CHAPTER 17 | *The Illness of Medicine*

before even adequately digesting the first one, which was mine. My less financially successful patients, however, generally seemed to accept their diagnoses more easily. Perhaps they didn't want to show emotion. Perhaps they saw cancer as just another hurdle in a life filled with them. Perhaps I just misinterpreted them.

The "anger" stage of grief is a very difficult one for the physician to manage. The anger is related to the perceived loss of control and to the fear of what the future will bring. It was during this stage that affluent patients would typically subject me to the opinions of their many family "experts," who would seem to come out of the woodwork and who, I was assured, were people of vaunted status and accomplishment. It didn't matter what their field of expertise was. One might be the chairman and CEO of Totally Irrelevant Incorporated, but he would call and inform me of his opinion. I would then be expected to hear the opinion of *his* closest friend, someone who'd attained even dizzier heights of accomplishment. This was a challenging time to be the physician giving the bad news. Often, I was told (in late-evening phone calls) of the myriad alternative treatments available, which patients would have discovered after scouring the internet looking for answers. In a few hours' worth of web research, the patients would learn the words, but they could never quite get the meaning of the vocabulary they now employed with such confidence. It takes years in practice to understand the ramifications of various cancer treatments.

If the patients decided to stay with me and not go off to some far-fetched treatment plan they'd heard about from another source, we would begin the bargaining stage of treatment options. Again, somehow the more access to money a patient had, the more complicated (often) the management. The wealthier were used to being in charge, and that's what they intended to be. In some cases, this behavior would lead either to their demise (as they traipsed around the globe in search of a miracle cure) or to their coming full circle, as they belatedly realized that no magic cure existed. The treatments I offered in Chicago were quite contemporary. I never forbid a patient to seek alternative care, and always recommended the patient to seek another opinion. But in many instances, the manner, the tone, with which the patient informed me of his or her getting another opinion was laced with contention. It was a choice each one had, and I felt obligated to recommend the standard of care, which had been vetted by many patients and practitioners long before my patient had ever had to learn about or deal with cancer. And in fact, some unusual, advanced, or complex cases did mandate that we employ alternative or somewhat more aggressive treatments.

I recall one particular patient who had sought an alternative treatment for his prostate cancer. In addition to the prostate cancer, he'd also been diagnosed with a rather severe gastrointestinal cancer discovered while undergoing staging (the process of evaluating the degree to which a cancer has spread). And yes, he did remarkably well. But his progress was highly unusual. His chosen treatment was not one I could recommend, despite his good results. Diseases, like most dynamic events, follow a bell curve, and there will be outliers at each end of the curve. I felt compelled to follow the consistent findings of clinical trials and to practice

CHAPTER 17 | The Illness of Medicine

guidelines buttressed by years' worth of research and review. If one wanted to seek alternatives, he was advised to be wary of treatments that sounded just too good to be true—particularly those with advertised rates of success that were conspicuous to the point of being suspicious. Cancer patients can be desperate, and some will latch onto whichever snake oil is marketed best.

The "depression" phase seemed to be short-lived. Given that most of the malignancies I treated were in men, perhaps it seemed this way to me simply because most men—once a treatment decision is made—want to get the damn thing started and over with.

Treatment for cancer can generally be divided in into three categories, and on occasion some combination of the three. The treatments are broadly surgery, radiation, and medical (which could include chemotherapy, immunotherapy, and hormonal or biological agents).

Which treatment modality is utilized depends upon the type of cancer, its grade (severity), and its staging (how far it has spread). Certain cancers are exquisitely radiosensitive, meaning they respond quite well to radiation. Others respond to a particular type of chemotherapy. Most recently, significant advances have been made in immunotherapy. Often, patients will come into the office with a preconceived plan of treatment based upon a friend's experiences. It is important to understand that one person's cancer is not necessarily comparable with another's. There are nuances to the type of tumor, aggressiveness, and stage that can influence how the cancer is best managed. In this difficult clinical situation, it is wise for the patient not to try to be the doctor at the same time.

Michael J. Young, M.D.

In my experience, the "acceptance" phase of cancer diagnosis and treatment involved a prolonged period of time. Patients would not "accept" their cancer therapy until they had moved past the other stages (anger, denial, etc.). But much of the outcome of cancer treatment is assessed over months or years. Also, how one assesses those outcomes is shaped by the type of treatment a patient has undergone. For instance, if a patient underwent surgical removal of his prostate, and the cancer had been successfully eradicated, I found the follow-up evaluation and blood testing (of prostate-specific antigen, or PSA) to be less traumatic. Patients who underwent radiation—another standard treatment, but one in which the prostate gland is left in place and then subjected to radiation—would also come in for testing. With the prostate still in place and producing PSA, slight variations in PSA levels would on occasion be identified, and these variations tended to cause anxiety. Although a curative state had been obtained, the radiation group of patients did appear to experience more follow-up worry than those who'd had their prostates removed.

Even in cases where cancer treatment is deemed successful, there's still the need to address the aftermath and the possible collateral damage caused by the treatment. How well a patient recovers, regardless of the *cancer outcome*, is influenced partly by such matters as the age of the patient and any comorbidities (other medical problems) that may exist. Pretreatment discussions of these secondary outcomes must be based on honesty, with the treatment accordingly tailored to the patient's needs and degree of understanding. I felt that the most important part of surgery was

CHAPTER 17 | *The Illness of Medicine*

never the surgery itself, which I knew mechanically how to do. The hardest part of surgery was making the decision *to do* the surgery for a particular patient. Before going ahead with any procedure, I had to confirm that the patient understood the *implications* of the surgery. Those who did were more likely to accept the outcomes and were more able to deal with possible complications. Nobody comes out of major surgery, radiation, or chemotherapy the same as they went in. Side effects occur, and all patients should assume that some aspects of their lives won't be exactly the same as they were before the treatment. Any reassurance to the contrary simply isn't the truth.

But the post-treatment phase of cancer intervention is when the most difficult development of all—recurrence—can occur. When it does, the emotional toll can be harder for the patient to bear than were all the previous stages of grief. This is also, obviously, the most difficult time to be the treating physician. The patients are understandably distraught. They'd been so relieved to be over their treatment, and had been hopeful of success. They'd been making plans to go forward in their lives. Events that had previously been put on hold were subsequently being put back onto their calendars. Patients at this stage feel that they already paid their dues, and any bad outcome is generally not tolerated well. Upon hearing the news of a cancer recurrence, patients are thrown back to the beginning of the grieving process, there to face for the second time all the frightening challenges they'd hoped were behind them for good. But with time and many discussions, patient and physician must move forward to the next level of therapy, however unbidden.

Michael J. Young, M.D.

And so it went in my own practice, cycle after cycle for the thousands of cancer patients I treated, who came into the office at various stages of cancer progression or regression, and with whom I faced the ups and downs of treatment success or failure. Most challenging, but also most important, was managing patients' self-perceived view of success or failure as they worked through the issues of their clinical status.

This was difficult work. It mandated a significant amount of emotional Teflon coating to prevent the daily events from being absorbed into my own personal mental space (an area that I think only a few patients fully appreciated). It was hard to do, and I was not always successful in separating my patients' outcomes from my own personal well-being.

I developed a very special relationship with many of my cancer patients, and over the years established close friendships with some. One of the common themes in these relationships was the respect we came to have for one another. Along with the significant problems they were facing, they understood that I was doing the very best I could to be forthright and empathetic with them. I would always advocate for them, and they recognized that. Whatever frustration or anger they experienced along the way, I never felt these moods were directed at me. These were resilient people. I admired their ability to stay focused enough to continue to work, to take care of their families, and to go forward with life. They fought hard, and I did the best I could to keep them in this process.

CHAPTER 18

The Incentive For Payment

There used to be a time when primary care physicians would try to treat whatever came into their office. They actually prided themselves on being able to take care of their patients without the need for a specialist. As medical outcomes have become the focus of greater and greater litigation, however, there's been a corresponding increase in not only the volume of referrals to specialists but also in patients presenting at earlier stages to these physicians wanting their problems resolved as soon as possible. Primary care physicians have become hesitant to treat a problem unless the condition is completely within their bailiwick. Similarly, patient intolerance of less-than-perfect outcomes is becoming more of the norm.

What is happening today is another twist on this situation. Toward the end of my days in practice, I was called by an internist who had a patient with a red, swollen penis. I was summoned from an exam room for this "urgent" call, and had to stop whatever I was in the middle of doing with my own patient to go to my private office and provide consultation. A description of the situation: A twenty-five-

CHAPTER 18 | *The Illness of Medicine*

year-old patient had had a red, swollen penis for the past several days, and the physician wanted a recommendation as to which would be the appropriate antibiotic. When I open my "Doctor Book" to the page on "red, swollen penis," I wish an immediate answer popped up to the effect of, *Difficult to make a complex diagnosis over the phone with a limited description of the problem.* There isn't just a particular antibiotic to be given to cure this "problem," because in a diagnostic sense, swelling and redness aren't root problems—they're signs, of something that remains to be determined. I don't know if I was more upset with the internist's attempt to make the problem so simple or with her failure to understand just how far from simple the situation and its treatment were. She was clueless as to the potential severity of the problem.

When a penis is red and swollen, possible explanations for this vary widely, and a careless diagnosis can be consequential. Maybe it's nothing more than a contact dermatitis, a localized reaction to, say, the rubber in the waistband in the patient's underwear. Maybe the patient has a cellulitis, a potentially serious infection that may turn develop into a life-threatening necrotizing fasciitis (a very serious infection mandating immediate surgical intervention, aggressive use of intravenous antibiotics, and hospitalization). Maybe the patient has contracted a sexually communicable disease. The internist was getting obviously frustrated as I explained the myriad reasons that could account for her patient's red, swollen penis. She wanted an easy fix-it pill.

I could not see her patient that day, since I was leaving town later that day and my office was already overbooked (for instance, "emergency patients" who'd failed to show up when previously instructed, now had to be seen), so I recommended that she send the patient to the emergency room to be seen. Most hospitals have a mandatory call roster, with call duty rotating among the various specialists. The system allows for coverage of or consultation on the various medical problems that come into the ER but that might be beyond the current ER staff's ability to treat.

The internist, however, pushed back, saying that she really didn't see the need for the ER, despite my informing her in precise detail how the patient with the red, swollen penis might have a significant problem. He needed to be evaluated and treated by someone with experience, and I was simply unable to take the case at the time. I had doubts that even the ER physician would know how to properly treat the problem, but at least the ER attending would contact the urologist on call, who I knew would see the patient. The internist persisted in arguing that an ER evaluation was unnecessary. It didn't seem to occur to her (or she didn't care) that since she didn't know what she was dealing with in the first place, she was in no position to make pronouncements on the validity of an ER referral. I wished her luck and returned to the exam room. By now my office was bursting at the seams with patients whose appointments had been delayed.

About a week later, I attended a hospital staff meeting. These were quarterly meetings that allowed interaction between the medical staff and the hospital administrators. Common topics of discussion were current events at the hospital, problems that needed to be addressed, and financial situations affecting the hospital. That

CHAPTER 18 | *The Illness of Medicine*

meeting's presentation was by the CFO, who was going over reimbursement changes.

Many of the primary care physicians' practices were owned by the hospital. Hospitals (or perhaps it's better to say the corporations that own hospitals) offer primary physicians a sum of cash for their practices and then pay the physicians a salary for their work tending to patients. This arrangement relieves a physician of the administrative and financial responsibilities that come with running one's own practice, responsibilities that include the hiring and firing of employees, the purchasing of equipment and disposable supplies, the managing of payroll, etc. Doctors generally don't possess good business acumen. With the years of medical training, few had exposure to formal business experience or education. Many feel it's a good decision to sell their practice to the hospital so that they can get back to the business of taking care of patients. Unfortunately, the arrangement contains a significant stipulation: the physician is no longer his own boss. He marches to the orders of the corporation that now controls (owns) him. Under the arrangement, physicians' salaries are determined by the hospital. This also means the physicians' office billing is calculated by the hospital/corporation. And guess what? The number of patients a doctor refers to the emergency room is monitored and tallied.

Now I understood why the internist was so reluctant to send her patient to the ER for treatment. Although she didn't know what he needed for treatment, she *did* know that an emergency room visit would be noted on her personal record of monthly or yearly metrics. This in turn would affect how her bonus would be calculated. She was being urged, by her employer, to minimize her ER referrals. If she didn't comply, there was a price to pay: her income might be affected.

So, what about the M.D. who doesn't sell his practice to the hospital? How does he function?

The answer to that question is becoming increasingly complicated. To own and run your own practice is becoming less common. The days of the doctor overseeing his own practice, with perhaps his wife helping, are dying out. Without the hospital covering everything from office expenses and malpractice insurance to increasing rent and rising labor costs, the private practitioner is forced to see more patients in less available time. Medical malpractice insurance premiums are at an all-time high. Perhaps the costliest budgetary development in recent years for those running their own practice has been the mandated use of electronic medical records (EMRs). The EMR was an inevitable development in the high-tech world in which we find ourselves. Doing away with paper charts and files offers obvious space and storage advantages, and being able to access patient records day or night has facilitated care. But the cost of these systems is exorbitant. Practices must pay not only for the software itself, which can top fifty thousand dollars per doctor, but also for the technological assistance, service contracts, and hardware necessary to connect the office. Given the decrease in insurance and Medicare reimbursement for nearly every patient encounter and procedure, more must be done in less time to keep ahead of such costs.

CHAPTER 18 | *The Illness of Medicine*

As a consequence of such budgetary distortions, private practitioners are now required to squeeze all they can out of the system, and not always for the right reasons. Basically it means they must see as many patients as they can, since time is money.

I was called one Friday at midnight by the ER regarding a patient with a relatively small kidney stone. I was told that the patient was in severe pain—no fever, no evidence of acute infection, just severe pain. With kidney stones, there are several criteria used to determine the potential need for hospitalization and/or surgical intervention. If a patient's pain cannot be managed, or if the patient can't hydrate himself due to severe nausea, or if there's evidence of infection or compromised kidney function, then hospitalization most likely occurs, and—just as important—insurance coverage for hospitalization is *approved*.

This particular patient had a stone three millimeters in size (roughly twenty-five millimeters are in an inch), and about seventy percent of stones this size will pass spontaneously—that is, without the need for surgical intervention. Probability of passage aside, the pain from passing even a small stone can be excruciating. The ER physician wished to have the patient admitted to the hospital, and asked if I would be on board for continued management. The patient did not report having a primary physician on staff at the hospital and was otherwise healthy. I agreed, gave the ER staff admitting orders and planned to see the patient first thing the following day.

During my morning rounds, I found the patient sitting up in bed, with a huge smile on his face. He had just passed his stone, and looked happy with himself, as though he had just climbed to

Michael J. Young, M.D.

the summit of a mountain. He proudly showed me his trophy-stone, now stored in a little specimen container, where it couldn't cause him any more discomfort. He looked fine and felt fine and desperately wanted to go home, as it was early Saturday.

Together with the patient, I reviewed his findings and the probable reasons for his kidney-stone occurrence, and then made follow-up plans. I wrote the orders for discharge and went on my way. It was around 8:00 a.m.

At 5:00 p.m., I received a call from his primary care physician, who was now making his hospital rounds. I'd never been informed, by the patient or the ER, that the patient even had a primary. This particular doctor was a private practitioner, with no hospital employment or oversight in play. He was incensed. How dare I send "his" patient home without giving him the opportunity to perform an examination? For that matter, how dare I even admit one of his patients without notifying him? I explained, patiently, that the ER had requested admission and that I didn't know why the doctor hadn't been notified. I also informed him that the patient never even mentioned that he had a primary. With each passing minute, the decibel level of the doctor's voice increased. He exclaimed, literally "patients do not fall from the sky," and said that if I ever wanted another referral from him (I don't think I had ever even seen any of his patients), I needed to understand how things worked. After taking his verbal thrashing, I regained my composure and inquired as to why he wanted to keep a patient in the hospital for the entire day, after the patient had obviously passed his stone. (I explained that I'd seen it myself in the little

CHAPTER 18 | The Illness of Medicine

cup.) The idea of keeping a patient in the hospital on a Saturday for an additional nine hours, to contribute absolutely nothing to the patient's condition, was beyond my comprehension. But I was then enlightened.

The physician could bill for the hospital visit. "Are you kidding me?" I responded. I was not only disappointed but dismayed as well. Is this what medicine had become? This doctor had the audacity to want to keep a patient in-house all day, for no obvious medical reason, so that the doctor could charge $100 for "evaluating" his patient.

So, these were the two extremes I faced in my private practice. On the one hand, there were the physicians who were encouraged not to send patients to the emergency room, and on the other, there were those who would keep their patients in the hospital for as long as they could simply in order to charge daily fees. I felt I was constantly walking a tightrope, wanting to do the right thing but having to balance that against what the medical system was encouraging, if not demanding. It was just a mess. The doctors had lost control of their domain. Medicine was now controlled by the corporations, by the insurance companies, and in some cases by sheer greed. For me, it was time to get out of this "business." This was not what I wanted and not what I had signed up for. I had gone to medical school and spent years in residency to learn how to take care of medical problems and patients. What I was witnessing was the detrimental influence of money in medicine.

CHAPTER 19

Fearing for Humanity

One of the mainstays of the urological management of bleeding within the urinary tract is to irrigate the bladder with fluid. This is not a new concept in resolving problems of contamination, and is often compared with the idea of "treating pollution with dilution." Also, when a patient is presenting with the problem of blood in the urine, irrigation may assist in allowing the urologist to isolate the source of the bleeding. Few things will scare patients more than seeing bright red urine coming out when they urinate. In my experience this situation causes more alarm in men than in women. Women have seen the effects of blood from their menstrual cycle. They have seen and felt blood clots occur. Although blood in urine is obviously from a different cause, the female reaction is still typically more subdued.

Men, however, with good reason, are much more agitated. Seeing blood come from the penis can be frightening.

The bleeding source can be anywhere in the urinary tract—the kidneys, the ureter, the bladder, the urethra, or the prostate gland. When bleeding occurs in the urinary tract, the urologist will need to identify the cause, often through a series of tests that will include imaging (CT scan, intravenous pyelogram, ultrasound, or MRI) and cystoscopy (looking into the urinary tract with a lighted scope). In the time between when a patient presents to the physician or the emergency room and when the cause is identified, the bleeding must be controlled. If it were to continue, the blood would eventually coagulate. When coagulation occurs, blood clots can often be seen in the urine, and if large enough, they can actually block the urinary tract and cause urinary retention.

One of the means of controlling bleeding that has led, or can lead, to urinary-tract blockage is to place a catheter into the bladder via the urethra to allow the bladder to decompress and drain. The goal is to keep the bladder from damage caused by overstretching, particularly if the bladder is the bleeding source. Similarly, if either the prostate or the urethra is the source of the bleeding, a catheter in place may have a tamponading effect on the bleeding site—that is, the catheter may help by putting pressure on the area of bleeding. If the bleeding is persistent, however, blood clotting could occlude the catheter. In that event, urologists may choose to irrigate, or flush, the catheter with sterile saline or water, to help remove the clots. Should the bleeding be even more significant, a particular type of catheter may be utilized, one that allows for continuous bladder irrigation (CBI). In this situation, a bag of irrigating fluid (sterile water or saline) is hung, much like a bag of intravenous fluid, with gravity causing the fluid to enter through a separate channel within the catheter. By this means, inflow and outflow are maintained without pause. The irrigating fluid is constantly instilled into the bladder, and just as constantly drained out through another, larger channel within the catheter.

CBI is extremely useful for managing significant bleeding of the urinary tract. With constant flushing, obstruction of the drainage catheter is minimized and the bladder is simultaneously kept at a constant low volume. As with all interventions, CBI requires diligence from the nursing service, in this case to ensure that the irrigation bags don't run dry and that the catheter urine-collection bags don't overfill. If either of these situations were to occur, the flushing would stop and the bleeding/clotting would likely recur. Often, CBI will need to run for days until the bleeding is reduced (as healing of the bleeding source occurs) or until the patient is stabilized enough for endoscopic/surgical intervention. It can be timely, costly (with charges related to nursing time and to the extensive use of sterile fluids), and potentially quite uncomfortable for the patient.

Illustrative of my increasing concern with some of the changes in the quality of physician training, I have a vivid recollection of being paged on a Saturday afternoon by a medical resident regarding an older patient who was in the hospital for a cardiac condition and who, during his stay, had developed urinary retention. He could not urinate. Often this occurs in hospitalized older men with enlarged prostates, and is attributable to prolonged recumbence in hospital beds, the use of various medications, as well as other concomitant issues.

CHAPTER 19 | *The Illness of Medicine*

The patient I was called for more or less fit this profile. A catheter was already in place, draining clear, yellow urine.

The page I received from the resident was regarding the use of CBI.

Ordinarily, when paged about a nonissue, in this case the resident inquiring if we should start CBI, I would state the obvious: "No. There is no need for CBI in this case. Thank you. Goodbye." That explanation was not sufficient for the resident during this conversation. She wanted clarification as to why no CBI was being performed. I strained to understand her, as it was painfully obvious English was not her native language. In fact, I wasn't actually sure she was even speaking to me in English. After several minutes of adjusting to her heavy accent, and while still not sure that I knew what she was saying, I seemed able to piece various portions of the conversation together. This could have been a skit on a television show. Unfortunately, it was real life. Her question, I gathered, was that if bleeding were to occur, should CBI then be started? I again asked if the patient was bleeding. Her answer, again, was no. Given that, I replied, why would she want to start CBI? This circular discussion lasted well over five minutes, though it felt like a lifetime on a lovely Saturday afternoon. All that time, I still could not figure out why I was being paged for a nonissue. There was no bleeding—not now or yesterday, and for no particular reason, I didn't foresee it occurring the next day, either. But she was fixated on having this discussion about what might happen in the future, and if bleeding occurred, whether she should start CBI. We went around and around.

Michael J. Young, M.D.

This is where I started to lose it. Realize that during a weekend on call, a physician can be bombarded with inquiries, complaints, patient worries, and bona fide emergencies—day and night. To be called by a physician in training who insists on discussing what could happen in the future, when there are no actual indicators that such an event will or is likely to occur, can be infuriating—the more so if this discussion in conducted in two languages, one being English and the other something else. Not only was she misunderstanding the nature of the problem (I tried to give her detailed instruction regarding urinary-tract bleeding and the use of catheters), but she was unable to understand even the words used to describe the problem. Utterly frustrated, I told her that if she represented the state of our medical education system, then I "fear for humanity." Typical of the conversation up to this point, however, my insult was completely lost on her. She even thanked me for letting her know the patient did not need CBI. There was never any question he did!

I think it's tremendous that students from all over the world come to the United States for medical training. It affords everyone a broader perspective, and introduces us to additional considerations for treatment. We can all learn from each other. But how can we have people emerge from our medical education system and enter into practice in our communities (people who undoubtedly take tests well, and pass exams) who can't actually speak the language of the communities they serve? Given the current state of medical practice, which involves less in the way of direct patient-physician interaction than ever before, I have significant concerns. What little

CHAPTER 19 | *The Illness of Medicine*

patient-physician interaction there still is mostly occurs while the doctor, with his back turned, types away on his keyboard. And as appointment time is increasingly being handled by midlevels and nurses, doctor-patient communication will approach perilous nonexistence if physicians don't have the skills necessary even to *talk* with their patients in the few minutes they spend together. Being capable of communicating in English, our official language, shouldn't be optional for a physician practicing in the United States. It must be mandatory. There is just too much at risk.

My misadventure with the non-English-speaking resident didn't even involve an emergency. Things might have been so much more consequential if it had.

CHAPTER 20

Responsibility

One of the issues I encountered as a surgeon was a nagging feeling of responsibility.

Going off to college at the ripe age of eighteen, I had no idea what lay in store for me. In college, your only real responsibility is to yourself. Once you decide what your focus of study will be, the classes you are required to take within that field of study are already determined. You decide whether to show up or not, and how much or how little to prepare for the required examinations. In college, most of your time is spent deciding what you want to do and when you want to do it. The responsibility for your successes or failures falls on you. Weekends in college could be spent catching up or letting go. It was dealer's choice, and you were the dealer.

Progressing in medical education slowly chipped that autonomy away. In medical school during the pre-clinical years, there were no elective classes. Taking the rough equivalent of forty hours' worth of classroom instruction a week, it was a constant struggle just to keep up with the required reading. "Free time" was a luxury few medical students enjoyed or controlled. During residency, long

CHAPTER 20 | *The Illness of Medicine*

before any limit had been placed on the number of hours a resident could work per shift, you worked until you were told it was okay to go home. Sometimes I would spend consecutive twenty-four-hour days in the hospital, working well more in that time than many do in a week. I was constantly exhausted. We were given two weeks of vacation a year. But I was sure things would get better, and that I'd be more in control, once I completed my training. It was merely a matter of delayed gratification.

But I was wrong. One of the things that, at the beginning of my residency, I took to be the mark of an "important" doctor was later revealed to be a noose around his neck: the pager.

Once I received my first pager, life was never the same. During my chief year of residency, we were no longer expected to remain in the hospital for night call. The year was 1990. The use of cell phones was still limited to the few who could afford them. Cell phones were still on an analog system (offering sporadic coverage at about thirty cents per minute), and most phones were the size of a brick.

Having a pager meant I could no longer have peace of mind, no longer go for a bike ride or even a short walk without a plan for how to get to the nearest phone as quickly as possible to answer any pages I might receive. Being at a teaching hospital, my fellow residents and I were paged for most everything. Being on call meant basically having a tether that controlled you night and day. It came with the territory, and I accepted that. Still, despite the hardship (or even because of it), the pager was worn or carried as a badge of importance, a sign of social standing. As I entered private practice, in 1991, I was in a group that covered a large suburban

Michael J. Young, M.D.

area in the northern part of greater Chicago. Again, I found myself being paged frequently—not by the nurses so much anymore but, rather, by the patients. Somehow, they had a funny way of defining what an emergency was. I learned that an "emergency" was really anything that applied to *them. Now!* There was no regard for the time of day or even consideration given to the appropriateness of calling at midnight. If a thought or question crossed their minds and they wanted feedback, well, they called. And they called. After all, I was their employee, right? Or so it seemed.

I often reminded myself of the contrast with what being on call was like in my father's era. He practiced medicine before pagers were standard. But more important, he was practicing when most patients had a level of respect for the physician on call. No patients telephoned at midnight simply because they were constipated, couldn't sleep, or because they had a burning curiosity about something. They called during regular business hours for such matters. And when they did call at night or on weekends, it was with an apology for the intrusion. Responsibility, in those days, was a two-way matter, observed by both patient and doctor. Somehow, that sense of mutual respect and obligation has been lost in our present "me-now" attitude.

Advances in wireless telephone technology tremendously increased one's freedom from the landline. Reliable cell technology allowed for days on call to be spent out and about, not merely indoors or within a short radius of a landline. Physicians on call were now part of the living world and could cultivate a more normal lifestyle.

Sort of.

CHAPTER 20 | The Illness of Medicine

There is no doubt that the mobile phone has changed all our lives. We go about things differently because of the freedom to communicate instantly from almost any location.

But phone access is just part of the equation. When I was on call, I still had a twinge of anxiety as I went about my day. Not so much because I felt that I wouldn't be able to handle the problem that arose but, rather, because I didn't have the choice to accept or not accept what was pending. Whatever I was doing at the moment would need to be suspended while I tended to someone's emergency, whether that emergency was real or not. Despite my desire to be in charge of my life as a physician, a surgeon, someone who made decisions that others acknowledged and followed, I had a responsibility. And with responsibility came sacrifice. This is something I wished patients had taken into consideration before they called at 10:00 p.m. on a Friday to change their appointment for the following Monday. Or before they called on a Sunday to discuss the "little pain" in their back . . . that had been there for two weeks.

Seriously.

CHAPTER 21

The Legal Mess

Whatever happened to the time when if you had a medical problem—say, if you stepped on a nail or had a persistent cough—you contacted your doctor, were treated, and went on your way. Perhaps that concept sounds rather 1950s-ish, but it worked. Let's look at such a scenario today.

You step on a small nail. It was stupid to walk around barefoot in the street. You know it, but you did it anyway. Fine. It hurts—not all that bad, and the bleeding has stopped, but you know it needs to be treated. You put your shoes on, finally, and get yourself to the emergency room. After the extended wait, watching others with more-serious issues being called in ahead of you and observing children climbing the walls out of boredom, you are called. Your vital signs are taken. You explain to the nurse how stupid you were. She nods with empathy, but is thinking to herself what a moron you are. Who walks around in the street without shoes on?

After a barrage of medical questions—including, at least four times, the one about whether you are allergic to anything—you again sit for what seems like ages. The doctor comes in and looks at your

CHAPTER 21 | *The Illness of Medicine*

foot. He gives you a sympathetic expression, and thinks to himself what an idiot you are. They thoroughly wash and then properly examine your foot. You are recommended to have a tetanus shot and an antibiotic. "You're not allergic to tetanus, are you?" The nurse asks before giving you the shot.

You are good to go. Well, not quite. Enough papers need to be filled out to equal a whole tree's worth of wood. Essentially, the hospital ER is having you sign and acknowledge medico-legal disclaimers stipulating that if your leg falls off because of the treatment you received for your stupid injury, the hospital is not liable. It doesn't matter that you were the one who foolishly walked in the street barefoot; that you created the problem; that you, the nurse, and the doctor all agree what an imbecile you were. At this time, you can sue the doctor, the nurse, and/or the hospital if your leg falls off (or is even somehow less than exactly what it was before your mostly self-inflicted incident). Despite your stupidity in causing the problem, they are now potentially responsible for what happens after their treatment. Medical malpractice is a booming business in our country. Were they negligent in their treatment? No, the right steps were taken to manage the problem. If your leg falls off, was it due to treatment on their part, meaning did they, cause it? Probably not. Was their care inconsistent with medical standards. No.

So in all likelihood, should a problem occur with your leg or foot, it might be difficult to find fault with the ER. Obviously, I'm not an attorney, but from my perspective, we don't have courts of justice. We have courts of law. It isn't just a matter of the *facts* that occur during a medical encounter. It is also a matter of what you (your attorney) can persuade a jury to believe. How well one attorney can outmaneuver another is really what matters. But during the legal process, the treating physician must endure not only the emotional trauma of the accusation of malpractice but also the significant costs required to defend himself. The time and energy spent meeting with a defense attorney are considerable, and the effort spent reviewing and preparing the documentation of events being questioned is exhausting. The mental anguish caused while ruminating over the episode is draining. The stress of the depositions can be absolutely painful. And at the end of deliberation, of consideration, the outcome of the legal case does not necessarily depend on what actually occurred. It depends on whether the jury *believes* a deviance in treatment occurred.

I had a middle-aged patient come in for an evaluation for urinary retention. He couldn't pee. This occurred after an inguinal hernia procedure. The retention was eventually resolved, and on a later follow-up visit, I obtained a PSA (prostate-specific antigen) test, which is used to help screen for the presence of prostate cancer. His test was abnormal. I called the patient to inform him of this finding and to recommend that we repeat the blood test and examination. He agreed to do so, but never came back to the office. Being concerned, I repeated the call, and eventually sent the patient a certified letter regarding my recommendation. The return receipt never arrived, so I sent another certified letter. Again, the receipt never came back. So I then sent the patient a FedEx, thinking maybe he didn't want to sign for any certified mail. Eventually I had proof of delivery. Fine, I did my due diligence by informing him of his potential for a malignancy. Just as important, I did what I thought was necessary

CHAPTER 21 | *The Illness of Medicine*

to *protect myself*. Why should it have taken two phone calls, two certified letters, and a FedEx; time and money spent because the patient was either too naive or too irresponsible to take care of himself? Yet I knew that if he were to claim I did not inform him of his need to repeat a blood test, he could find an attorney to sue me.

I experienced two lawsuits filed against me during my years in practice. The first was related to a patient I had seen in the office for what sounded like a kidney stone. The patient was a semiretired, part-time security officer around seventy years of age. He came in stating he had some intermittent, mild flank pain, with blood in his urine a month earlier. At this time, he was feeling well without any complaints. His physical examination was basically normal, with the exception of his being obese, yet he did have microscopic amounts of blood in his urine. He had no flank pain, and no abdominal masses could be felt. I recommended to him that we begin with an x-ray of his kidneys to try to find out what was going on. At that time (the early 1990s), one of the x-rays utilized for evaluating blood in the urine, and identifying if a patient had a kidney stone was called an intravenous pyelogram (IVP). CT (computed tomography) scans are now the imaging procedure of choice. During the IVP, radiocontrast is injected into a patient's vein, and after the blood is then filtered by the kidneys, the contrast shows up in the urine. Given that the contrast is radiopaque, the excretion of the urine in the urinary tract can then be visualized on x-ray film. The patient was given a prescription for the x-ray and was to return in several days. There was no emergency presenting, and the patient was symptom free. Unfortunately, three days later,

Michael J. Young, M.D.

while I was on vacation, he came to the hospital emergency room for what was now significant flank pain. Around the same time that he came into the ER, a massive auto accident occurred on one of the main expressways in Chicago, with over a hundred cars involved. Given the consequent influx of traumatic injuries into the ER, the patient was assigned a lower status while the more acute trauma victims were given priority. Nonetheless, his pain progressed, and after several hours he got his IVP exam, as the ER staff also felt that his pain and recent medical history were consistent with a kidney stone.

The films came back verifying a three-millimeter (relatively small) kidney stone that was now in his ureter (the tube connecting the kidney to the bladder). Size does not correlate to the degree of pain caused by the stone. Small stones can be just as painful as large ones, and the pain can be overwhelming. Female patients told me over the years that childbirth was less painful than passing a kidney stone.

So the patient had a kidney stone. But as the ER staff was still tending to trauma patients, he was relegated to a less prioritized section in the emergency room. His pain continued and then worsened. Consequently, the patient's blood pressure rose, eventually topping 220mm Hg (normal is approximately 120mm Hg). He then blew out an abdominal aortic aneurysm (AAA). The aorta is the main artery in the body. Should there be a weakness in the wall of this vessel, or a large enough aneurysm (a bulging of the vessel), the aorta is susceptible to rupture. As the patient's blood pressure reached dangerously high levels in response to his pain, this may

CHAPTER 21 | The Illness of Medicine

have contributed to the rupture. With his sudden deterioration, the patient now became a true emergency, as acute as any of the trauma cases currently in the ER.

By the time the rupture was identified and he was rushed into surgery for treatment, it was too late. He never recovered, and subsequently died.

I returned from my vacation to hear of these events. Although I had only met the man three days earlier, he was deemed "my patient," and consequently I was sued for not knowing he had had an abdominal aortic aneurysm. Not that I, or anyone in the ER, could have felt an AAA on examination, given the patient's obesity. Furthermore, his x-rays and IVP never revealed any abnormality or calcifications consistent with his AAA.

It was an unfortunate event. The exquisite pain from his stone probably caused his blood pressure to elevate and this, feasibly, contributed to the aneurysmal rupture. Had this happened at home prior to any doctor visits or ER evaluation, his death would not have become the subject of a lawsuit. Given that he presented to the hospital for a kidney stone, however, and despite appropriate evaluation, the fact that he had had an unknown aneurysm was now everyone else's fault. It didn't matter that the patient hadn't had his blood pressure regularly checked, or that he'd rarely seen a primary M.D. routinely in the past, or that he'd been obese and in poor overall health. His family's lawyer initially named some twenty individuals in a legal suit because of this event.

Michael J. Young, M.D.

I went through two years of agonizing review and depositions. It was a horrible time of self-criticism. I would see nearly a dozen patients a week with the diagnosis of kidney stones. I was being sued because this particular patient, unknown to me, had had a kidney stone *and* an AAA. Was I now to send all new patients I saw in the office for kidney stones immediately to the ER for evaluation, even in the absence of pain or physical abnormality on exam? At that time, CT scans were not yet routine. This man's case was unfortunate, but was it my fault? No.

After two years of maneuvers involving insurance companies and legal firms, I was dismissed from the case. Tens of thousands of dollars had exchanged hands as a result of the process. Sadly, the patient had died. But hadn't he or his family had any responsibility for his health and his failure to avail himself of more regular medical care? Apparently not.

The other malpractice case I was named in was just ridiculous. A chain-smoking alcoholic had had a hernia repair. He was having trouble urinating postoperatively, so I was called in to evaluate him. Other than his inability to void his bladder and the usual postoperative incision findings, his exam was normal. His urinalysis was normal. A catheter was placed, and then removed several days later, after his activity improved and his postoperative pain had been minimized. He left the hospital urinating fine. Despite being given discharge instructions for follow-up, he never returned for urological evaluation. Two years later he was diagnosed with bladder cancer. Despite his smoking (a well-known, significant risk

CHAPTER 21 | The Illness of Medicine

factor for bladder cancer) and despite his forgoing the recommended follow-up, he and his lawyer felt it appropriate to sue me because of his cancer. They claimed I should have known about it from his urinary retention two years previously. Really? How?

Once again, after months of legal back-and-forth the case was dismissed. Even the personal-injury lawyer the patient had hired eventually realized the absurdity of the suit and its high likelihood of failing in court. There would be no quick settlement and easy money for the lawyer on this case. It was simply another frivolous suit that caused significant angst for the physician involved in taking care of a patient's problem.

Why should physicians tend to a patient's problems or complaints if at the end of treatment, a suit is filed because of an undesired outcome? Why, is the patient's responsibility for his own condition rarely taken into account? The patient is free to smoke, drink, and do most anything he wants, secure in the knowledge that he can blame someone else for life's untoward events. There is something drastically wrong with our society if this is the new mainstream philosophy.

The eagerness of personal-injury lawyers to go after an undesired life event—seemingly regardless of their client's responsibility, regardless of lack of factual corroboration for the lawyer's contention—has polluted the legal system. In order to proceed with the lawsuit, the malpractice attorney needs a "medical expert" to agree to the validity of his case. Often, the actual legitimacy of the expert himself is a question in and of itself. Until the law is changed to stipulate that court costs and everyone's legal fees will be the responsibility of the plaintiff should the court rule in favor of the defendant, frivolous cases will continue to be filed. Given our current legal climate and our society's distorted perspective on personal rights versus personal responsibilities, many a committed, dedicated physician will soon call it quits. Who will be left for you to call when you or your family experience an emergency? Not I.

CHAPTER 22

Building A Practice

During my urology residency, a combined six-year process, the residents were expected to complete two years of general surgery, followed by four years of urology training. During the first two years, the resident was exposed to a variety of surgical situations: general surgery (for instance, colon, hernia, and gallbladder surgery); vascular surgery (repair of diseased blood vessel); plastic surgery; ear, nose, and throat procedures; trauma services; and so on. The urology training was specialized, dedicated to learning how to treat such conditions as infertility and erectile dysfunction and those related to neurologic urology and urologic oncology, and to cultivating the skills needed to perform such things as reconstructive urology and endourology.

Teaching at all levels has been a doctrine of medicine since the beginning of formal medical education. The intern taught the medical students, the senior residents taught the juniors. All of us took it upon ourselves to ensure that the next-in-line would have acquired the skills and judgment necessary to carry on the work.

CHAPTER 22 | The Illness of Medicine

I clearly recall being a chief urology resident mentoring an intern who had just joined our service. She was a young intern who was still considering surgical options for a career, and she was drawn to the adrenaline rush of trauma care. The acuteness of the situation, the life-or-death decisions that have to be made over a matter of minutes, the thrill of a successful resuscitation—all can be intoxicating to a young, newly minted M.D. She elected to leave her spot in our program and go into trauma surgery as her specialty. Sometimes, it's hard to counsel new, young surgeons on what lies ahead. They think they know all.

After completing my training, I elected to go directly into private practice. I wanted to be self-employed, to hang my shingle. For my practice to succeed, multiple events had to occur.

First, and most generally, I needed to make myself known to the medical community, to get the word out that I was willing and able to treat urological conditions. I needed to make myself available to other physicians for referrals in my specialty, and I needed to assist some primary care physicians with how to evaluate normal urological health. I also needed to provide medical education and awareness at community discussion groups, churches, and firehouses. I would offer myself to any and all. It was hard, tedious work. It required so much time and effort to "remind" the referring doctors that I was available. There was always a bit of reluctance on their part to trust their patients to the new guy, an unknown quantity. After all, a bad outcome from surgery would reflect badly on *them* for having given the referral.

Second, I needed to demonstrate affability, prove that I was a "good guy." In order to develop a relationship with referring primary care physicians, I needed to schmooze them, be part of the inner circle at the hospital. This meant spending my free time in the doctors' lounge, being around to listen to others' jokes and laugh when expected (regardless of how bad the jokes were), all to gently remind the other physicians of my presence. There were already established urologists on staff, and they protected their referral turf. But as the new guy, I had two advantages: I was well trained in the most up-to-date surgical methods, and I was willing to take on problems that other urologists didn't want to spend time with. I would take the chronic problems that couldn't be billed as much as a new, acute condition. I would take any public-aid patient that others had declined because of the low reimbursement involved.

Finally, if most obviously, I needed to demonstrate ability, making sure that my surgical cases went smoothly and that my complication rate remained low. In order to successfully demonstrate this in the beginning stages of my practice, I had to be a bit clever and selective. Although I'd been trained in complex urological surgery—of the sort that might involve entry into the chest, the abdomen, and the pelvis, sometimes all three in the same procedure—I chose to limit myself to the more basic surgical procedures during that first year in practice. I didn't have enough standing among my newly acquired referral base to effectively weather a bad outcome. I worked to build a stellar reputation, not one of excuses for why things hadn't turned out well. Later, after having established myself and my practice, I could risk complications without fear of losing future case referrals. I then took on the bigger, harder cases. Timing is everything in life.

CHAPTER 22 | The Illness of Medicine

The three *A*s of developing a successful private practice: availability, affability, ability. In that order.

Eventually, through hard work and long hours, I built a strong, solid practice. My referral base was broad, and I had an excellent reputation. Most gratifying—and telling, I felt—was the devotion of my patients, who continued to come to me for treatment and evaluation. But this success certainly didn't develop overnight.

Years later, as I reflected on why I had chosen my field, I had occasion to recall that young doctor in my program who'd left urology to go into trauma care. I was exiting one hospital emergency room on my way to another hospital for rounding, thinking of how complicated some trauma surgeon's day was about to become. A code yellow had been announced on the hospital intercom, an indication to staff that a trauma victim was inbound and would soon be presenting to the ER. In early residency, these calls were the highlight of training. Dealing with gunshot wounds, vehicular trauma, and severe sports injuries of all sorts was undeniably exciting. But when you're a resident, there is always someone behind you to call, to summon, to rely on for experience in managing critical situations. As an attending physician, there is no one to turn to for the unexpected conditions or complex issues you are facing. You are the end of the line, and it can truly be a daunting experience. For the attendings who specialize in trauma, they are on their home turf. But that turf wasn't mine, so as I heard the intercom buzzing with the news, I was glad to know I was not on call for that problem, that particular day.

As I arrived at my next hospital stop (specialists are often on multiple hospital staffs), I heard another crackle on the intercom: a code pink

Michael J. Young, M.D.

from the intensive care unit. A code pink is an elopement. Did a patient really just get up and leave the ICU without being noticed? A patient who undoubtedly had multiple intravenous lines, perhaps a urinary catheter in place, and however many other measuring devices attached, just got out of bed and eloped without notice? Another day of practice. Another day spent in a hospital.

I had built the practice I wanted . . . but where was it now going? I enjoyed what I did. But the daily grind was starting to wear me down. How many nights could I go without sleep? How many evenings were to be interrupted by calls from frantic patients? I could bring them down from their panic, after years of experience doing so. But I was having trouble bringing myself back down into my own world. The thoughts of what had just been discussed during each evening or nighttime call from a patient were lingering longer, interrupting my own rest and respite from the office. The weekend call schedule was becoming more demanding as well. I had residents available to go to the hospital for consults, but the patients were ultimately my responsibility. Residents were still physicians in training, and their evaluations and recommended treatment plans required verification.

Many of my colleagues not only *asked* the residents to see their patients and consults on weekends, but depended on them doing so. I felt that as the attending physician, however, I was the one being called to evaluate a problem. So I would go into the hospital frequently at night and on weekends. This was fine when I was younger, but it became increasingly difficult as I entered my second decade of practice.

Eventually I brought partners into my practice, which was growing and becoming difficult to handle alone. I still wanted to offer the

CHAPTER 22 | *The Illness of Medicine*

same care, and I trusted my new partners to carry through with my work ethic and values, yet I never quite felt that the partners shared my vision. But then, I had *built* the practice, whereas they reaped the rewards of its already having gone through the stressful startup phase. The process of receiving referrals for new patients was much easier for them, since the referral base had already been tirelessly built with years of lecturing and follow-up calls and hours of curbside consults on my part. I'd invested significant worry and sweat in that time. When my latest associate joined the practice, the patients and their surgeries were already lined up for him. He had less anxiety about doing enough work to pay the rent, pay the staff, pay for office supplies, and still make a living. So much had already been done.

I wasn't thrilled with my partners' way of going about things. They relied more heavily on the residents and midlevel care providers than did I. This appeared to be a pattern in other practices with younger associates as well. Perhaps it was a consequence of my own compulsion, but I never felt that the partners were seeing patients in the hospital as regularly as I was. Maybe such frequent rounding wasn't necessarily medically indicated, but again, recalling the three *A*s of a successful practice, two of the three, availability and affability, were paramount. As a consequence of their less frequent hospital presence, I heard rumblings from referring attendings. My partners just didn't get it, and I suspected they never would.

The successful practice that I'd nurtured—with devotion, time, and energy—was becoming less recognizable to me. I did not want to question others' priorities anymore. Perhaps the time had come to start considering retirement.

CHAPTER 23

Meeting in the Doctors' Lounge

I had just arrived in the doctors' lounge to begin my Sunday-morning prerounding ritual, which involved making a cup of tasteless coffee in the semiworking coffee machine and trying to find a doughnut left over from the day before, and maybe a banana if I were lucky. I was on call for our group: Friday-through-Monday coverage. Most calls during such shifts were not urgent, and involved things like recurrent urinary-tract infections and questions regarding surgery from the previous week. Occasionally, however, a serious call came in involving a truly sick patient, a urologic trauma case—someone who needed immediate surgery and attention.

The previous day (Saturday), I'd been called in the morning by a patient who had undergone a percutaneous nephrolithotomy performed by one of my partners several days earlier. This is a procedure in which a large kidney stone is treated with the placing of a tube through the skin (*percutaneous*) into the kidney directly, whereafter the stone is fragmented and removed utilizing either ultrasonic or laser energy (*nephron* refers to kidney; *lithotomy* refers

CHAPTER 23 | *The Illness of Medicine*

to surgical treatment of a stone). The patient was complaining of constant vomiting and chills that began earlier in the night. I recommended that the patient come to the emergency room, which he did within an hour of our discussion. I met the patient and his wife. They were both frightened. In the ER, the patient was in a septic (infected) condition. He had tachycardia (fast heart rate), sweating, and chills and a high fever. He was uncomfortable, with significant flank and abdominal pain. Subsequent imaging showed no obvious kidney blockage from the stones that had been treated. However, his condition was consistent with a diagnosis of pyelonephritis—an infected kidney. This is a nonsurgical condition that calls for intravenous antibiotics and treatment of the vomiting and fever with aggressive hydration and antipyretics (fever reducers). The patient was admitted for continued monitoring and care.

As I was preparing my coffee on Sunday morning, and about to head up to the medical floors to make rounds, I ran into an internist in the lounge who wanted to congratulate me on my upcoming retirement. He asked why I was hanging it up at such a young age. I explained to him my frustration with the state of medical care. We discussed my disappointment that hospital care was being delegated by many primary practices to the residents and hospitalists. Hospitalists are hospital-employed physicians who see hospitalized patients in lieu of the patients' being seen by their own primary care physicians. Many hospital systems or practices, in order to increase productivity, stipulate that in-house patients are seen in this manner. Hospitalists generally have no knowledge of or prior interactions with patients who are now not only in need of medical care but also in need of a friendly face, that of someone they feel they can trust in their time of illness. A patient may have been seeing his regular doctor for twenty years. But suddenly, when he is in the hospital, rather than being treated by the person he knows, he's instead under the care of the hospitalist. Such management, as dictated by the hospital/corporate structure, improves "efficiency," and now—often—the primary care physician is limited only to outpatient or office visits with his patients. Some primary care practices, were a hybrid in their management of in-patient hospital care. In these instances, the primary would come in during his or her on-call weekends.

* * * * * * * * *

The internist I saw in the lounge nodded in solemn agreement. Yes, he said, it is truly a shame that the patients are now being seen and treated in such an impersonal way. The care is so splintered, and the primary care physician is often no longer directly involved in patient care once hospitalization occurs.

Apparently, he was on call for his group that weekend as well, and while preparing to make his rounds, he studied the computer screen in front of him. I surmised that his group took over on the weekends for the hospitalists. It was confusing. Care was just so divided up that often, as in this case, I wasn't quite sure who to call when I needed to speak to a primary. Who was covering for whom?

CHAPTER 23 | *The Illness of Medicine*

The internist asked me if I knew anything about a new patient on his list, a patient admitted the day before with pyelonephritis. He knew nothing about the case, and as he tried to read his new patient's name properly, I was stunned. The septic patient I had seen twenty-four hours previously in the ER had been admitted to *his* service, apparently without his knowledge. Even though this internist would be tending to his group's patients during the weekend, I felt he should have been aware of the patient's presence and status. The baton had been passed to him now, without apparent appropriate communication.

With that, I began to lose my sense of politeness. How could he be responsible for a patient that had been in the hospital, under his name and service, without his having any knowledge of the patient's condition or status, let alone the admitting diagnosis? It appeared to me this patient had been treated like little more than a name on a spreadsheet that had turned up in his inbox.

But, he assured me, unwittingly justifying the very system he and I had just been complaining about, the residents would of course call him if they felt the patient were in trouble. But how would they necessarily know? Residents are students, and the intern on his service was only four months out of medical school. And, of course, the hospitalist overseeing the residents, hadn't informed him in the first place of the patient's admission. Nonetheless, the doctor felt "quite confident" that if the patient fell ill, he would be notified. I reminded him that this was exactly the problem we'd discussed, the one behind my decision to get out of practice, the one that involved a lack of concern, a lack of supervision, and a complete disregard for doing what is best for a patient. The one that said trust the junior physician (resident) to treat, and to call if problems arise. But how could anyone expect a junior resident to have the ability to know if a problem was looming?

The doctor realized the weakness of his position. In calling out the system of care, I was essentially calling out his lack of care. He expressed his displeasure by gathering his papers and exiting the lounge.

Did I make an impact on the internist's understanding or appreciation of the problem? I think so. I think deep down all capably trained physicians know what is supposed to be done for patients. And they know that indifference and a loss of direction both need to be addressed.

Years ago, when I operated on a patient, I would call the internist to update him on the procedure and would usually get in reply an inquiry about how the patient was doing. Today, I am instructed not to bother the internist in the office, since he or she is busy trying to meet a mandated patient quota. Instead, I am to call the hospitalist. I call the hospitalist. He doesn't know the patient from the man in the moon. It's highly unlikely he even met the patient before surgery. The hospitalist's first question is rarely about the surgical outcome, about how the patient is doing. The hospitalist's first question, almost invariably, is "When can the patient go home?" Seriously.

"Well, let's see, Doctor," I want to say, "the patient you are now 'covering' lost two liters of blood during his six-hour cancer

CHAPTER 23 | *The Illness of Medicine*

operation. Maybe he can go home in thirty minutes. Will that meet your efficiency guidelines and financial criteria? He'll be one less patient for you to stop by and see. You can check his name off your list, without ever having to learn anything about him." Such are my sour thoughts. Is there a bonus or incentive for getting patients out of the hospital sooner? And if so, who is monitoring this and how is it being monitored?

I detest the hospitalist system. Yes, there are of course some very fine physicians who have chosen this career. However, in my opinion it encompasses all that is wrong with health care delivery today. Primary care physicians are put under significant financial pressures and time constraints by the hospitals or corporate systems that own their practices. These doctors are spinning like mice on a wheel to move patients, people who have paid a lot of money and expended considerable resources for quality health care. These patients are being cycled in and out as quickly as possible. The doctors and everyone else in their office are mostly typing away at their computer terminals, documenting a lot of crap—not necessarily treating the patients' problems efficiently, or even effectively. But the corporate, hospitalist system mandates that they perform at a pace geared to generate one desirable, quantifiable outcome: Revenue.

CHAPTER 24

Nobody Can Do Anything

I witnessed a significant deterioration in the ability of many physicians to handle interventions in any fashion other than to call someone else to do "it." Over the last decade or so, my attitude progressed beyond the point of being astonished at such inability. In the end, I expected nothing. When did this start, and who is to blame? Not infrequently, I found medical students and residents, young physicians in training, often averse, and therefore unable (for lack of practice), to perform any number of the rather basic medical interventions. And where did they learn their habits? Probably from the senior residents, or possibly even the attendings, who in so many ways encouraged them to "call someone." As the residents graduated—without having had the experience they should have had—they simply became attendings who were incapable of performing the most basic of interventional tasks, which they now, still, deferred to someone else. And the cycle of lack-of-proficiency continued. Obviously, as an attending, performing such tasks would not be routine, or necessarily appropriate. But the students and the residents, those learning their

CHAPTER 24 | *The Illness of Medicine*

craft, must be exposed to and be able to perform basic interventional techniques. It is part of learning the art and skill of what it means to be a physician.

* * * * * * * * * *

So, what do I mean? Well, let's start with the basics. My understanding of what makes physicians so special is not only their commitment to helping others but their willingness to try.

The practice of medicine in the general sense can be broken down into several categories. One would be surgery and its subspecialties (orthopedics, urology, plastic surgery, etc.). Another would be medicine in its various forms (internal medicine, family practice, pediatrics, etc.), as well as its subspecialty fields (pulmonology, gastroenterology, nephrology, etc.). And the third would be areas of medical practice that broadly apply to both (anesthesiology, radiation oncology, radiology, etc.). When I was in training, our goal was to learn as much as we could not only about our own fields of interest but about others as well. For example, we made daily x-ray rounds, which involved physically going to the radiology department, since digital imaging did not yet exist. We looked up the films of our patients, whether they were chest x-rays, gastrointestinal studies, CT scans, or ultrasounds.

We reviewed them as a group and would ask any radiologist passing by for help. Without fail, at any hospital, no matter what time of day or day of the week, were a radiologist available, he or she would be willing to help us. The radiologists wanted to help us learn. We wanted to learn. Today, things have changed. The radiologists are still there and willing to teach, but many students no longer appear interested in learning topics outside of their specific discipline. I guess it's just easier to call someone to interpret the imaging for you.

I saw medical residents who were barely able to discern a kidney from a bladder on imaging. Today, nearly all imaging is digital. Viewing the pictures can be done from any computer in the hospital and, with proper credentialing, from one's home computer as well. All one has to do is spend a few minutes actually looking at the picture to learn about the patient. But that basic curiosity has not been instilled in many of today's students of medicine. What numerous physicians have apparently learned instead is that there's no reason to expend the effort studying images when you can simply wait for the radiology report to come out.

I recall being consulted once to see a patient with gross hematuria (blood in the urine). The word "gross" implies that the blood was visible without any magnification. In other words, this person was urinating red, bloody urine. It is a common indicator of pathology in the urinary tract. Blood can be seen in cases of cancers (kidney, ureter, bladder, prostate, etc.), trauma, significant infections, or vascular anomalies (abnormal blood-vessel development) within the noted organs. On occasion, blood can also indicate relatively minor conditions. It is the job of the urologist to identify the cause and then establish a treatment to resolve the problem.

CHAPTER 24 | *The Illness of Medicine*

One of the basic tenets of troubleshooting hematuria is to evaluate the "upper" urinary tract first, namely the kidneys and ureters, and then asses the "lower" urinary tract, the bladder, prostate (if present), and urethra.

I walked into the patient's hospital room with the medical resident. The patient was in no apparent distress, and red-wine-colored urine could be seen draining from a Foley catheter. After I examined the patient, I discussed with the resident the plan for a CT scan and the subsequent need for a cystoscopy (a procedure that involves looking inside the lower urinary tract with a light-equipped endoscope). The resident proudly informed me that, indeed, he had ordered the CT scan upon the patient's admission. Good.

Did he look at it? No, of course he didn't. Not good.

I went on to explain to the medical resident how important it was that he look at all of his patients' x-ray studies. If he spent about thirty minutes a day doing this learning exercise (the films can be studied while sitting in a chair, drinking a Coke, and munching on pretzels), he would be that much better a physician. He stared at me in response as though I were from Mars. Apparently, nobody had ever stressed this to him as emphatically as I had.

Once he recovered, he told me that he was looking forward to finishing his internship year and moving on to training in his specialty, which was none other than radiology.

You've got to be kidding me, I thought. Here was a student of medicine, bound for a career in radiology, who was so uninspired, so poorly motivated either by himself or by his "teaching" supervisors that he didn't bother to look at the CT scan of this patient. That he ordered! His chosen field of study! The purpose of the internship is to see patients and *integrate* imaging, pathology, presentation, and management. That is, the purpose is to actually learn something about treating and managing disease!

Stunned at his response, I guided him by his proudly worn white coat the five feet to the computer monitor, *in the patient's room*, and together we looked at the CT scan. Having a radiology resident who is not interested in his own patient's scans should be unheard of, yet this was not just consistent with how inadequately he himself was being overseen by his more senior residents and attendings but was pretty typical of what I witnessed in today's training/learning in general. Not good, indeed.

I recalled my medical school clinical rotations and internship year, and the feeling I had on morning rounds after a good night on call ("good" meaning you had the chance to do and see a lot). I remembered that if my fingernails had blood under them, I knew I had been busy. We drew blood ourselves, we inserted nasogastric tubes (through the patient's nostril and down into the stomach to drain gastric contents), we placed our own Foley catheters. We did blood cultures and obtained arterial blood gases. This required obtaining blood from an artery, typically the radial artery in the wrist, and then running it down to the lab ourselves to measure blood oxygenation levels. We didn't call the surgeons or urologists for help unless—and only unless—after trying in earnest, we were unable to draw the blood or get these tubes into patients.

CHAPTER 24 | *The Illness of Medicine*

These days, it's not just medical residents who often won't make the effort to perform these rather basic medical interventions. On more occasions than I care to recall, a fair number of emergency room (ER) physicians wouldn't make the effort either.

EMERGENCY ROOM ISSUES

I worked with some truly outstanding ER physicians throughout my years in medicine. However, with increased regularity, I was called into the emergency room, at night, to place a Foley catheter, when the ER attending had not even attempted to do so. The excuse was usually something to the effect of, "Well, I'm just not very good at it, so why try?" Well, if the physician had tried years ago, he probably *would* be good at it now. As with anything, practice makes perfect (or better, at least). I could accept someone's trying and failing. But not to try at all, more out of sheer indolence than actual lack of ability, should really be an embarrassment to anyone calling himself an emergency-room physician. It's not appropriate to rely on the specialist as a matter of course, particularly when the procedure is one that should be within that specialty physician's ability. Just try! In my case, after having to run into the ER in the middle of the night to place a Foley catheter, I had to show up in the morning, on limited sleep, perhaps to operate on you, or your father, or friend. There are consequences to every action, or inaction.

ER physicians today are trained on most every organ system. They are taught the—presentations and initial management of trauma, of infection, of "plumbing" systems that have gone awry (gastrointestinal, pulmonary, urological). Obviously, they have a lot of territory to cover. Often, lately, it seems they ignore their training and focus instead on mastering the on-call list so that they can have the ER receptionist page the specialist at first sign of need. Certainly, there can be an emergency or a condition requiring specialty consultation. On far too many occasions, however, the calls were for things ER physicians should be able to handle without recourse to specialist intervention.

Even more annoying, yet increasingly common, were the midnight phone calls "just to let you know." The ER physicians had become so averse to taking even minute risks (ones inherent to the job) that they felt it necessary to inform the specialist of every detail, practically as it was happening. But at 2:00 a.m., does the urologist really need to know about the inconsequential one-millimeter kidney stone (quite small and likely to pass on its own) for which the ER is sending the patient home on mild pain medication, just so that the urologist can anticipate the patient's call for an appointment in the morning? Worse still, I witnessed patients admitted to the hospital for Foley placement for urinary retention, with the catheters still in their original packaging resting on gurneys, awaiting a urologist to place them when the patients were admitted to the floor. The ER physicians didn't even try! Foley placement is something that could have been, and should have been, handled in the ER, allowing the patient to go home without being admitted to the floor.

I also found that ER physicians were increasingly dependent on imaging. Once, for example, I was called for a patient presenting to the ER with the complaint of lower abdominal pain. I was informed

CHAPTER 24 | The Illness of Medicine

that a CT scan had been obtained and it revealed that the patient had two liters (2000 milliliters) of urine in his bladder (recall the size of a two-liter bottle of a soft drink). The average bladder will hold roughly 300 to 500 milliliters of urine. For reference, the volume of a soft-drink can is 355 milliliters. Did the ER staff really need to spend $1,000 to $2,000 of the patient's insurance money (or Medicare) to obtain this scan? Had they not considered asking the patient when he last urinated? Had anyone considered performing the increasingly rare art of physical examination, by actually placing hands on the patient's abdomen to note a peculiar bulge the size of a grapefruit right above the patient's pubic bone? When such queries were put to the attending staff, the excuse was, "We might have missed something."

Really? C'mon. Enough.

* * * * * * * * * *

Are these issues related to a lack of training? Sometimes. Lack of interest? Possibly. Medico-legal concerns? Certainly. There is no question that the medico-legal environment has caused a significant change in how we practice medicine. The over ordering of imaging studies and the overreliance on them for treatment are becoming all too common. And, of course, once the imaging is processed, rarely does anyone bother, because rarely does anyone have the confidence, to just look at the results for even a preliminary assessment. Everyone just waits for the official report. Some M.D.s would probably have difficulty identifying a baseball in someone's mouth without a CT report in hand, confirming that the round object keeping the patient's jaws apart is, indeed, a baseball. Actually, and all the worse, the official radiology report on this event would never be that definitive. It would read something like this:

Radiology Report re: object noted in patient's mouth. History obtained: patient was hit in the mouth with a baseball. "A round object is seen in the patient's mouth. Noted baseball-type stitching is appreciated surrounding round object. Object appears to have a cork interior. Possibly consider object to be a baseball. Must also consider other anomaly such as tumor of tongue or lips. Clinical correlation recommended. Would also recommend follow-up MRI or ultrasound for verification, or whatever other x-ray you didn't already obtain."

Good thing we now have radiological confirmation. Now we can proceed to carefully pull the baseball out of the patient's mouth—but first let's put on our mandatory two pairs of gloves.

In addition to x-rays, labs tests are often ordered superfluously, because of a lack of confidence, because of a lack of knowledge, or again, because of medico-legal concerns. I really don't think, in most cases, having blood drawn day after day after day in the hospital is productive. A patient's arms become bruised from all the needle sticks. It hurts, and it's also most likely not necessary—ordered more out of habit or the need simply to order something. But this is nothing compared with the possible long-term effects of exposure to unnecessary x-ray radiation. Let's think

CHAPTER 24 | The Illness of Medicine

more before (reflexively) clicking the box for more testing on the computer screen.

In urology, I had countless elderly men, older than eighty-five years of age, being referred to me because their prostate-specific antigen (PSA) tests, which are used as a screen for prostate cancer, were abnormal. And so they were, but what was the actual need for the test at this age? Probably very little, since most prostate cancers are slow to progress and would not be a factor in the remaining years of the average eighty-five-year-old patient's life. Many such patients would die *with*, rather than *from*, prostate cancer. So why were PSA tests being performed on this age group? Lack of knowledge, probably. I saw a doctor order a PSA exam for a ninety-five-year-old man on a ventilator, who was in the hospital following a cardiac event. A physician should know what tests are necessary and indicated. Physicians should take responsibility, learn what is necessary and what is not, do the right thing, and be accountable.

Yes, I understand the concern about legal entanglement. Every patient I operated on was a potential plaintiff against me. Indeed, in medicine every client/patient that you welcome into your practice can turn around and be your worst legal nightmare. But that is no excuse not to try to do your best. Patients are coming to you for help. I simply ask physicians, whatever their current status in training or in practice, strive to be exceptional. Do your best to espouse the privilege of being a physician.

CHAPTER 25

First Case, Last Case

I was so thrilled to walk into the operating room the very first time as an observer. I was so disappointed as a senior attending surgeon as I finished my very last procedure.

What happened in that interval? What had I seen, felt, and experienced to make me so disillusioned with the practice of medicine that I wanted to get out of the field?

Attitude.

But whose attitude had changed? Certainly, I was fatigued from the nearly constant pressure of having no margin for error. Concern over being accused of malpractice was and is always on the entire medical community's mind. How exactly had the practicing of medicine, of applying science to cure illness, become so subject to litigation that protecting against legal vulnerability became the main driver of a significant portion of our diagnostic testing and imaging? How had we, as a sophisticated, developed society, come to endorse such perversities as a need to find legal blame for unexpected or undesired outcomes? The inclination, and perhaps

CHAPTER 25 | *The Illness of Medicine*

even desire, to find fault when events don't turn out as wanted is deplorable. Aside from rare instances of actual negligence, in nearly all cases physicians want to do the right thing, and *do* do the right thing. Mistakes happen. Of course. But it's folly to assume that every medical outcome will be successful, and it's erroneous to define success as reasoned by the patient's attorney the only legally acceptable outcome. Such expectations, backed up by legal threat, have made a travesty of medical care. So many of the less scrupulous personal-injury lawyers take advantage of bad consequences and encourage finding fault in bad outcomes. Bad things can and do happen when we try to treat a bad condition. And yes, there are cases in which the doctor did not perform in a manner consistent with the standards of care. But how appalling are those plaintiffs who go after the very physicians who tried honorably, and with considerable effort, to make their lives better. As long as we have a society that feeds on blame, however, and have courts that don't make plaintiffs in frivolous suits who lose their cases pay all court costs and legal fees, the travesty will continue. Congratulations, America. You now are down one more competent, compassionate doctor to harass. And what if the litigious patient finds himself in need of a physician emergently one day, but none are around or willing to take the responsibility for his care? That's really too bad. The public has sued and harried them out of practice. Good luck with your pain. I'm sure someone, somewhere, with a false promise and some snake oil can help. Go sue them.

My tolerance for patients' lack of responsibility, or simple common sense, was diminishing. Yet, if they didn't seem to care about or pay attention to themselves, why should I be upset? Perhaps I was frustrated dealing with the unprecedented sense of entitlement so many patients were now exhibiting. They demanded swift resolution of their problem, regardless of any role they may have played by ignoring simple signs and symptoms for months or even years. Somehow, the complaints got louder while any expression of gratitude after appropriate treatment was all but nonexistent. When I started practice years ago, I would receive many well-wishes and thanks, in simple notes acknowledging the care I'd given. When I left practice, I found myself satisfied with an occasional "thank you" as someone walked out the door.

I will always remember the night I was on call and awakened at 2:00 a.m. for a testicular torsion. This is a true urological emergency. These events are excruciating for the patient and dangerous to the organ, and must be tended to immediately. The testicle receives its blood supply from the testicular artery, a branch off of the aorta, which is the main artery of the body. The testicular artery and venous structures, a network of nerves, lymphatics, and the vas deferens are bundled together in a "cord" that basically traverses the inguinal canal and descends into the scrotum. If this cord twists upon itself, sort of like a bell at the bottom of a chain, the testicular blood flow is diminished and the testicle can become necrotic. It will die within hours if not "untwisted." I rushed to the hospital and took the patient to surgery. I successfully remedied the torsion and finished the case at about 5:00 a.m., just in time for another day of work to begin—a full day of patients, problems, and surgery, possibly scheduled months earlier. Again, there are no mistakes

CHAPTER 25 | *The Illness of Medicine*

allowed in this business, no matter how much or how little sleep the surgeon has been "allowed."

The patient did well and came back for a postoperative evaluation a week later. His testicle was intact, and he was healing fine—so fine, in fact, that when I left the room momentarily to take a call, he slipped out of the office. There was no "thank you," and there was no payment, either. He had no insurance, and he made no effort to compensate me in any way for my effort, training, and expertise. Yet had he *perceived* that I performed the procedure incorrectly, or if the outcome had not been as desired, a personal-injury attorney would have assumed center stage.

Physicians are nothing but human. We remember these events. Being treated in such a manner would make anyone angry. It is insulting. Yet, if I were called the following night for the same problem, I would have dragged myself out of bed and done the best I could. It was all part of a commitment I'd made long before. But the grind was getting to me. Understandably, the daily problems all of us experience—jobs, family, financial stresses—plus, in my case, the discontent of dealing with a medical system in flux, made me question staying in medicine.

Perhaps patients had lost their willingness to put up with all the crap as well. Was it greed within the medical industry that was wearing them—and me—down? From my perspective, observing how some practitioners took care of patients, it was evident that the patient had come to be seen as little more than a conduit for financial gain. In practices that changed their business structure from a true partnership to one of individual billing for services,

Michael J. Young, M.D.

I saw an immediate ramping up of the volume of procedures performed. Any communal, democratic spirit that had previously been obtained seemed to go out the window once independent billing became established. Some of my physician friends complained that in their own practices, corporate meetings had become more focused on identifying revenue streams than on evaluating medical treatments. I noted that in many instances, leadership positions were filled by those focused on quantity, not by those with experience or seniority. I felt the quality of medical care was waning, that the emphasis had shifted toward the profit motive and away from actual concern for the patient and his or her outcome. That shift was a mistake. The work ethic that resulted was not one that would enhance patient care.

Now multiply this perspective across all medical fields and across all practitioners. Physicians, too, were tired and frustrated with the increased pressures to meet quotas. At the same time, practice costs have increased. The costs of employee benefits, equipment, and rent have quadrupled over the years. The burden of student loans required for medical school has become nearly unbearable. And, of course, insurance reimbursement for services provided has continued to drop considerably. Meanwhile, the premiums doctors must pay for malpractice insurance, mandatory to allow them to practice, have only risen.

With all of the pressure to perform flawlessly, with all the energy required merely to navigate the bureaucratic minefield it was getting harder to come out at the end of the day fulfilled and happy with how I'd occupied myself. The considerable time, energy, and

CHAPTER 25 | *The Illness of Medicine*

effort spent improving other people's lives were taking a toll. In the beginning, successfully treating disease was a pleasurable challenge, but now practicing medicine was taking more out of me than it was giving back.

I trained for years to learn how to perform particular surgical operations exquisitely well. It was hard work, both mentally and physically. It required commitment and significant personal sacrifice (of time that might have been spent doing other, more desirable things). But being a surgeon, *a good surgeon*, meant being available to others. It meant being prepared to leave every weekend get-together or party. It meant being called away from birthday celebrations, anniversaries, and other personally important events. Things that seem commonplace become so precious and important when you can't participate in them due to concerns of having to run off to the hospital. To take care of patients, who in general were becoming increasingly entitled, and to do so in an increasingly hostile practice environment, was becoming difficult.

I enjoyed immensely the opportunities I had as a surgeon. I practiced medicine in an exciting, stimulating time, but that was years ago. Undertaking the surgical steps for each procedure—which I had worked so very hard to become proficient at, and to learn front, back, and sideways—had once been a rewarding exercise unto itself, but was now no longer gratifying. The anatomy and physiology, the biochemistry and physics, I studied along the way will always fascinate me. But the social *application* of science—medicine—had become so ensnarled as to be dysfunctional. The joy was gone. It was time to move on.

CHAPTER 26

Time to Stop

It is time to stop, time to take stock of what is happening in the practice of medicine.

If we want it to be a business, well, we are there. Pharmaceutical companies will continue to have armies of "reps" sell us their drugs, drugs that are advertised on television to an audience that has absolutely no idea regarding drug interactions and safety—unless you really think the thirty-second disclaimer in each advertisement is sufficient. The ads are insulting. Today, it seems every third TV ad is about a new drug you "should know about." I suffered through several television advertisements this morning as I was watching the news. A full-minute advertisement discussed a new drug for cancer treatment. Twenty seconds of the ad described the drug in such detail that even with a medical background I was unclear about the specific indications. The remaining two-thirds of the ad were composed of legal jargon and specified risks associated with the new wonder drug. Another ad I heard, equally confusing, described a new medication for diabetes. It went into detail regarding "HbA1c" values (a means of assessing blood sugar

CHAPTER 26 | The Illness of Medicine

levels), as though the average person watching the ad could *fully* understand what this lab value implies. No problem, viewers can just go to the internet and learn all about it in ten minutes. The drug companies give their web addresses during commercials just to make it that easy.

It took me years to understand the ramifications of prescribing medications in all their variety, and in those years I came to know how the drugs affect individuals. The mere notion of telling viewers to talk to their doctor about the latest purple pill is just absurd. It is a disregard of medical responsibility to suggest to a potential patient, without proper counseling or consideration of alternatives, that his or her condition can be remedied by the taking of a specific pill. These ads, by design, are akin to showing the leash to a dog. Suddenly that's all the dog wants, all he can think about—a walk, going outside. The patient now comes to the office *expecting* that drug seen on television, having been encouraged to seek this solution to his or her ailment. There is no television explanation given to the viewer as to *why* the problem may have come about, what its approximate causes might be—just swallow something and make it go away. Side effects? Viewers, while watching the ad, heard that part of the legal boilerplate about how they "may die" and how the company disclaims any responsibility in the event that they do. But will the drug really work? Dunno. Let's just get it and see.

What about the cost? I haven't once heard a television advertisement go into actual financial detail. The pharmaceutical company might hint at an offer to "lend assistance." But paperwork equal to that of a mortgage will need to be completed first, and then reviewed. And then probably rejected. Either the disease will have resolved itself or the patient will have succumbed to it by the time the review has been completed. And as for cost, again, why is the same drug so much cheaper in other countries? Business as usual.

* * * * * * * * * *

That corporations control the financing of much of the health care delivery system is a significant problem. Corporations will continue to buy medical practices and dictate to the physicians where, when, and how much they should practice. The physician is no longer in charge of his or her patients' health care delivery. He or she is told how many patients must be seen and in what time frame, and what interventions are "allowed." For instance, Disease X is to be treated by Pathway X, which has been determined to be the most cost-effective, or most financially profitable—depending on your perspective. Consequently, the doctor's office is no longer a health care sanctuary, a place to go for comfort and healing. It has become a monitored, managed, pathway for billing. The patient has become a mere triggering mechanism for unlocking the flow of money within the health care system.

The patient has a problem. He pays his copay. The insurance enterprise will request a referral from the doctors "owned" by the medical corporation, and treatment will continue down the

CHAPTER 26 | The Illness of Medicine

assembly line. It will plod along the preestablished path. The physician will perform treatment and follow-up care as he has been instructed to do. Most likely, his salary and bonus depend on his compliance with the corporate system objectives.

If the patient selects a doctor who is not within his or her network, then a small battle will ensue. The physician is simply trying to treat the problem. The patient's insurance company, however, is attempting to mandate that the least-expensive, but not necessarily the best, path to resolution is followed. X-rays and other tests will undoubtedly be challenged by the medical administrator of the insurance company. The patient, who is already paying exorbitantly high premiums, is expecting to follow the treatment plan indicated by his physician. But he will be disappointed when he discovers that the treatment plan has probably been modified at the insistence of the insurance company.

Incidentally, why do banks and insurance companies seem to have the tallest buildings in the skyline? Just a thought. I suspect the "golden rule" applies: He who has the gold makes the rules. Maybe I shouldn't risk straining my neck by looking up so much.

Hospital administrators are no longer functioning simply as organizers of the facility. They are now also tasked with implementing the corporate goal of profit maximization. For example, they hire outside consultants and regard patient care as a very calibrated *business* decision. They assess the space available in a doctor's office and monitor room usage. They base the hiring of a new physician on a calculated appraisal of the profitability that may ensue. How the doctor's presence may enhance the hospital or clinic's image is an absolute top consideration. And if the doctor practices great medicine, well, that's good too.

I suspect a work-efficiency ratio that has been predetermined by the corporate hierarchy dictates the actual amount of time a physician is "allotted" per office appointment. But how can some outside consultant, probably without any direct or even indirect experience in understanding the ramifications of a particular disease or condition, start dictating to the physician how much time is to be spent per patient? Let's see the administrators come into the office accompanying a physically or mentally challenged member of their own family, someone who has difficulty understanding the nuances of his or her own problem. Let's see the administrators' reaction as we try to professionally and ethically treat their loved one "by the clock." Unfortunately, this thought-provoking scenario is unlikely to occur. Usually, whenever a hospital VIP needs an appointment to be seen, the red carpet is rolled out. I doubt very much that their needs would ever be subject to efficiency models and standard practice.

I can remember being at surgical department meetings where the focus was on the actual minutes each surgeon spent on a particular case or procedure. The results had been tabulated, and the surgeons' names were lined up on a PowerPoint slide for everyone to observe: "Minutes per case." From a pure business perspective, it was a measurement of productivity and efficiency. But the patient on the table, rightly, wishes only that you take the time necessary to resolve his problem properly. He doesn't want to be a statistic in a quarterly earnings report. It's easy to stress the primacy of time management

CHAPTER 26 | The Illness of Medicine

as long as it's someone you don't know or care about who is having the operation. Accordingly, it's the obscure insurance companies that ultimately collect data on time management and then use the findings to "encourage" hospitals to increase efficiencies. To a certain degree, I believe, contracts to hospitals are dependent on these and other nonsensical metrics.

I understand efficiency. I also understand outcomes. If I were the patient and had a physician who was slower than most but had stellar results, I would go to him without hesitation. I don't want the doctor who prides himself on speed. True success is measured not by the clock in the operating room but by the quality of the results. I have seen painfully slow surgeons who also have painfully bad outcomes. Obviously, this is not desirable. But the measurements of success the hospitals appear to be emphasizing are speed and efficiency, and such misplaced priorities will contribute to bad outcomes. I'm quite sure hospital administrators and organizers would deny that this is what they're doing. They would reply with shock and dismay at the assertion, insisting that *of course* patient safety and quality outcomes are their highest concerns. And to a degree, I believe that's true, but they also insist that you ensure safety and quality as quickly as possible. Time is money, both in the office and in the OR.

I recall at one of the hospitals, the administration spent tens of millions having a consulting firm assess the efficiency of the hospital workflow. The consultancy dispatched "experienced" twenty-five-year-olds to monitor the floors and observe the interactions among the nurses, doctors, and patients. These young consultants made their recommendations after about three months of being in everyone's way, and their plan for workflow overhaul was absolutely moronic. Not one of these consultants had a clue how to organize what was necessary. A hospital is not a factory. There is no production line. There is no product at the exit. There is a human being with a problem, with a family, a job, a life. There are short- and long-term goals for recovery. The concept of managing health as if it were a widget to be produced is just ridiculous.

* * * * * * * * *

We live in a society of medico-legal absurdity. As I drive along the freeway, I see one billboard after another with some scholarly looking medical-malpractice attorney gazing down on the passing cars. No money is charged unless "you" win, the billboards promise. What a wonderful system. Why not sue somebody because you have lung cancer? It wasn't your fault that you smoked despite all the warnings. Not to worry—the malpractice attorneys will try to find someone to blame. I have seen ads promoting lawsuits for nearly every known cancer, as well as birth defects. These attorneys will sue whomever they can "on your behalf." Yet whenever I meet one of these liability lawyers, they all claim they "don't take just any case—only the real cases." Right. Contemptible. Most really don't care about your medical condition. I suspect they care only about how much profit your condition can earn them.

CHAPTER 26 | *The Illness of Medicine*

In parts of the country, malpractice attorneys have sued so many neurosurgeons that there now aren't any neurosurgeons available when neurological emergencies actually occur. What a shame it would be if one of those attorneys' family members fell off a bicycle and struck his or her head on the pavement—and suffered irreversible damage for want of proper care. It would be genuinely tragic. Is this really the type of health care availability we want in our society? If you want to sue, go ahead. But our laws need to change. The plaintiff and possibly his attorney (who dangled promises in advertisements) needs to bear responsibility if they lose in their accusation of malpractice. The current free-for-all to anyone with a grievance, but without any consequences for filing a frivolous allegation, is simply wrong.

* * * * * * * * * *

So how do we go forward? What mechanism for changing the course we are on can be implemented to facilitate better health care? We have the best technology on the planet. We also have the greediest health care delivery system. As long as individuals and entities—physicians and their employers, pharmaceutical and insurance companies—strive to make outrageous profits from health care, caregiving will continue to be warped toward that end. And yes, again, everyone from practitioners to medical administrators to pharmaceutical executives insists that patient safety and health outcomes are their main concern. But no—it's a competitive business, and patient outcomes are not what they are selling. Yes, I think on some primordial level they do want the patient to get better, but if they can make some money along the way ... And therein lies the trap.

There are many very fine physicians truly dedicated to delivering the absolute best care. They have studied for years, and they do their very best, for all the right reasons. They will stay up all night. They will work until near total exhaustion takes over. These devoted health care workers will do their utmost to ensure that care is delivered as well as it can be.

Unfortunately, I have found that this type of physician is becoming extinct. More realistically, many newly minted M.D.s will typically work shorter hours, be less available, and spend more time typing their exam results into a computer than they spent on the examination itself. The young doctors will probably expect more time off, have more shared responsibility, and will deliver a more predetermined, preplanned course of treatment.

Until we cease thinking of health care as a business and see it instead as a means of addressing a predicament—a predicament that in one form or another, at one time or another, will affect us all, something we all must share and accept as equals—we will not improve our health care delivery system. Until the business of medicine is removed, and the actual *practice of medicine* is again the priority, we are destined to continue on this path of dysfunction.

CHAPTER 27

How Do We Get Out of This Mess?

How did health care reach this breaking point? Was it because of the corporatization of medicine and the influence and entanglement of the insurance industry? Because of greed among physicians? Because of laws that attorneys have crafted both by and for themselves? Because of all of the above, perhaps?

There is no doubt that the influence of those who control the purse strings has been a major determinant. Hospital administrators work for a boss. Whoever owns the hospital controls those who administer the ownership's directives. Today, many hospitals are owned by a corporation. The corporation, whether a for-profit entity or a so-called nonprofit, is still mandating that mechanisms be in place to ensure a surplus of earnings. In a capitalistic system, profit is key. However, in the medical field, we are not building or selling a manufactured product. We are tending to human health and well-being. Patients shouldn't be viewed as shoppers forced to shell out for wellness and, literally, in some cases, their own lives. Using the maintenance of those most basic necessities of health as a means of reaching a desired profit margin is the source of the problem. Many hospitals are now implementing various

CHAPTER 27 | *The Illness of Medicine*

measures that may provide a service but also significant income, often an exorbitant income. When measuring the success of a hospital, quality outcomes must be chief among the considerations. But in my experience, quality was often considered secondary to such measures of success as speed, volume, and efficiency. In countless hospital meetings, quality outcomes were discussed only *after*, say, the number of minutes of operating room used and the number of patients seen had been thoroughly scrutinized and measured against established efficiency quotas. Admissions, discharges, length of stay, are understandably important business metrics. But my concern is what is driving these analyses, and how the data that is obtained is really being used.

As previously noted, I have seen hospital administrators turn slightly away in sheepish acknowledgment when a particular surgeon is mentioned, one who brings in a lot of work but whose outcomes (at least from a health standpoint) are less than desirable. They know he is at best mediocre. No way would *they* go to him for treatment, but the hospital just lets the surgeon continue to operate. Often, the hospital will do so until the whisperings about his lack of ability become too audible, or a tragedy occurs. Then there is an administrative uproar. Action is instituted with a flurry, and the hospital makes every effort to show publicly its dismay and shock. But the corporation made huge profits because of this surgeon, before cutting him off.

And what happened along the way to bring this surgeon to such an end? When he was fresh out of medical school, he was enthusiastic about medicine and probably wanted to make a difference. He had studied hard and worked diligently to achieve success in his field. What was it that eventually turned him into a money-making machine? He had a skill set that prompted referrals. People came to him for help, and he had an ability or a technique to accomplish what patients needed. One possible explanation is that his costs had gone up. He had built too large of an office. Expenses had increased, and he had too many mouths to feed. Perhaps his lifestyle had become too lavish. But I suspect differently.

I suspect part of it was a sense of entitlement. In this surgeon's view, he not only had worked hard but had also *sacrificed* himself. He had given up too much along the way, and now he would claim his compensation. I surmise that in the early days he performed a procedure quite well, and then realized the monetary potential, at which point the boundaries determining when and whether to perform the procedure began to blur. Soon, more procedures were being done, and an increasing number of them were of dubious need, performed on patients whose presentation would not have led to a recommendation of surgery by other surgeons. Consequently, more avoidable complications occurred. Having weathered a few of the complications with his reputation intact, the surgeon was emboldened to undertake yet more questionable surgeries. The cycle continued, and widened well past the limit of safety and appropriateness. Only if disaster occurs does the cycle stop, at least momentarily. Until then, the surgeon and his hospital or surgical-center employers keep happily adding up the numbers on the bottom line.

CHAPTER 27 | *The Illness of Medicine*

Someone is paying for all of this. Name any insurance company. It doesn't really matter. Hospitals will negotiate with different insurers, who will then "allow" their patients to have their health care covered at a particular institution. Certain hospitals, despite possibly having outstanding reputations, may not be on the "preferred" list of a particular patient's insurance. Consequently, a patient will be "directed" to another facility for care, one that might be farther away or otherwise less convenient. It doesn't seem like an onerous situation, unless you now need to drive two hours or so roundtrip each day for your outpatient radiation treatment (over a duration of two or three months), or need to do so merely to visit an ill parent. Not only do insurance companies determine how much they will pay for an insured patient's care. They dictate where that care is to be delivered.

They are paying the bill, so essentially they can determine outcomes. Perhaps your insurance provider has a relationship with your doctor, meaning that that doctor is on the list of referring physicians you are allowed to see. Good. But perhaps the physician most qualified in your area is not on the list. Tough. It doesn't matter that you are paying an absolutely exorbitant premium and have a deductible seemingly large enough to pay for a new car.

The insurance companies control your access to health care. As a patient, you have limited status to negotiate, reason, or cajole. My experience has been that even the most mundane of testing must be approved by them before you are allowed to get care for the ailment that the insurance actually covers. If what is required by your physician is not within the standard playbook (a playbook to which only the insurance company has access), you'll need your physician to contact the insurance company's medical director. And the position of medical director, as stated before, is occupied by a physician who typically, in my experience, sounded on the phone as if he or she couldn't care less. Many times, I felt that I was pleading with them. I rarely spoke to one who impressed me, or who had a significant understanding of the problem. I never once spoke to an insurance medical director whose comprehension of my specialty-related issue was equivalent to my own. Yet, the directors make the determination of what constitutes appropriate testing and treatment. The insurance company medical director is just another roadblock. (From the insurance company perspective, the directors are ensuring "quality and necessary care." No. From my point of care, they are containing company costs with whatever measure they can.)

So, the insurance company sells you, the prospective patient, a policy. It sounds good. It looks good on the TV ads, what with everyone jumping about in a park, feeling well. You obviously don't need the policy—until you do. And then you realize the company will dictate where you can go for treatment, which doctor you can see for treatment, and oh yes, which medications you're "approved" for—or not. If you choose "not," you will be forced to pay the equivalent of a monthly home mortgage for the medications your physician originally prescribed. The health care product that you desire, that you *need*, is now under the control and direction of the insurance industry.

CHAPTER 27 | *The Illness of Medicine*

So why is medical care so costly? With the all-knowing insurance industry managing so many aspects of your care, and with you paying through the nose for this care, wouldn't it seem to follow that costs are effectively being contained? Well, ignore for a moment that the insurance industry has CEOs whose compensation packages (salaries, bonuses) are huge. There are also the lobbying costs, paid by the insurance company. And how much does a one-minute television ad cost in prime time? No wonder the insurance industry has to charge so much. Look at its overhead.

Then there is the significant issue that physicians are practicing defensive medicine in order to shield themselves from liability. Physicians are, indeed, overtesting. Why? Because of the zeal for litigation in this country. And once again, to protect themselves from potential bankruptcy should a significant malpractice event occur, doctors need to pay exorbitant malpractice premiums to, of course, the insurance industry. It's one vicious circle. And who seems to be sitting right in the middle, directing the flow of medical availability, opportunity, and, of course, money? Yep, the Insurance Empire.

And whatever happened to the sacred patient-physician relationship? With all this concern for and emphasis on costs, payment, referrals, and copays (again, all dictated by the insurance companies), the actual confidential relationship between the patient and the doctor, which for years was considered a bedrock of dependability, has now been reduced to a regulated minutes-per-patient assessment on a spreadsheet analysis of productivity. Profitability and productivity have become the new chief measures of success in the medical industry, the most-desired outcomes, toward which hospital corporations and insurance companies push both doctors and patients. If a patient's health is restored in the process, well, that's good too. If not, maybe the patient can be referred to somebody else. Oh, "somebody else" is not in the patient's "plan"? That's really too bad.

Also, younger M.D.s are coming out of school with enormous debt. Subsequently, they are under significant financial pressure right out of the gates. Many have been trained in an environment that actually limits work hours. This affects subsequent working expectations and can limit the doctors' ability to experience a continuity of patient care, which is mandatory for understanding a disease process and its possible directions. Many times, I felt an indifference from them while I expressed trepidations about my patient's progress or condition.

The residents also spend more time typing into an electronic medical record than they do examining any given patient. The structure of medical care now enforces scrupulous documentation and a strictly limited appointment schedule. The system has beaten them up as well. Their reimbursement is less and out of their control. They are frustrated, even angry, with what has happened to their domain. I have worked with many truly fine residents, who want to do the right thing for the right reasons. But they, too, are trapped in this seemingly unending deterioration of a contaminated system.

So, the lawyers sue, because they have been asked to do so by an angry, entitled society. Patients are frustrated by a health care

CHAPTER 27 | *The Illness of Medicine*

system that no longer values them but that responds, instead, primarily to the insurance industry. The doctors are angry with the loss of their sovereignty and their ability to control boundaries they spent difficult years trying to establish. And the central theme in all this chaos is the Control of Money in Medicine.

How the money in medicine is allocated dictates the care that we, as patients, receive. How it flows—how it is controlled and regulated—determines who gets what quality of care. To help get us out of this morass, the central role of *money in medicine* must change.

I understand the economic and organizational complexity of the medical enterprise. *Medicine* encompasses multiple, interrelated undertakings: research, education, supply and service businesses, and ultimately, the clinical treatment of an illness or disease. These interrelated undertakings, as a whole, make up nearly one-sixth of our gross national product, and affect nearly every aspect of our daily lives in one form or another. From the moment we awaken, we are applying, swallowing, inhaling, or utilizing some product of this vast realm. Successful treatment of disease could be considered one of the triumphs of our society. But we have allowed the finances encompassing medicine to control that treatment.

We as patients, unfortunately, have become casualties of the commercial greed that has attended the successful managing of disease. To fix this problem will require a change in our thinking about how we manage disease and illness. Should health care as an industry be controlled at the federal level? Should it be a single-payer system? If we eliminate the need for profit from all of the sublayers involved in medicine, and if we take out the quest for profitability, I believe the costs for care would decrease significantly. A baseline for care could be established, one that everyone, regardless of personal wealth, could expect to receive and wouldn't be required to "buy." If a wealthier patient desired a particular provider or healthcare facility, that would certainly be his or her option to pursue.

But the current health care environment, in which money is made while choreographing individual health events or misfortunes, is not sustainable. Until we recognize that we are *all* patients at one time or another, we will continue to go down this dysfunctional path. We must change our perspective. Health care is not a business but, rather, a priceless societal necessity. We must all work together with the same goal in mind: to cure the illness of medicine.

EPILOGUE

We have taken a look behind and around the process of health care delivery, from the perspective of both patient and provider. We examined and reviewed how one experiences medical treatment from both sides of the table. The significant obstacles patients endure, as well as the exasperation many of the truly dedicated medical professionals feel, has been assessed. The controlling arrogance of the insurance industry and the clout pharmaceutical companies have over us have just become overwhelming. I recall a time when these industries worked with, and for, us. Today, they appear to be the opposition. Patients have essentially no control, and doctors have lost the ability to direct their own profession. Profit-driven corporations dictate how our care is governed. This is an undeniable problem. We are all frustrated with how we are so restricted, so vulnerable as we struggle to navigate through our health care system. Most painful is how we are treated by the medical system itself. Absent today is the sense of concern and empathy we used to associate with the medical profession. We yearn to be treated with compassion; to have trust and confidence in those engaged in taking care of us. Unfortunately, *medicine* has become a mechanism of profit. It has become a business whose own bureaucratic tendencies have spread like a powerful, aggressive disease.

While working as a provider, I lost confidence in how our health care is delivered. Medicine is now structured by a system seeking maximum return on investment, with human health as its currency. For me, the joy of studying medicine, applying that knowledge, and helping someone in need had been overwhelmed by bureaucracy.

But I do think we can correct this path. As with any dilemma, the first step is recognition—open acknowledgement that a problem exists. My intent is that this book will help to open a dialogue between patients and physicians. Indeed, we are not on the opposite side of the table. Rather, we're on the same side. Every one of us will be in need of health care at some point in our life. We must recognize that the problems reviewed here affect us collectively, not just as individuals. We, both patient and provider, must go forward and confront the issues.

Assuming we recognize the problem and accept the need for change, how and where do we begin this process? With a communal push. And we should push hard.

Changes in health care delivery can occur. But the change we need won't be driven by the grievances of only a few. Nor, as stated earlier, will it occur quickly. It will require many voices, together, demanding a transformation of our medical system. But just as politicians can be made to sway to the complaints of their constituents lest they risk subsequently losing votes, so can the various managers within our health care system be pressured and directed. We must begin applying this pressure: challenge our employers for better insurance options, persuade our politicians with our elections, reiterate our complaints to health care providers and hospital/facility administrators, reassess what products we buy and companies we support. Doctors, organize and take back your domain from corporate control. We must have respectable health care, at a respectable cost, without manipulation and exploitation by the current business enterprises. With dedicated effort, we *actually can* make a transformation in how our health care is delivered.